LEARNING AND MOBILISING FOR COMMUNITY DEVELOPMENT

T0271868

Learning and Mobilising for Community Development

A Radical Tradition of Community-Based Education and Training

Edited by

PETER WESTOBY and LYNDA SHEVELLAR
University of Queensland, Australia

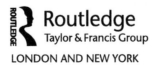

Routledge
Taylor & Francis Group

LONDON AND NEW YORK

First published 2012 by Ashgate Publishing

Published 2016 by Routledge
2 Park Square, Milton Park, Abingdon, Oxfordshire OX14 4RN
711 Third Avenue, New York, NY 10017, USA

First issued in paperback 2016

Routledge is an imprint of the Taylor & Francis Group, an informa business

British Library Cataloguing in Publication Data
Learning and mobilising for community development: a radical tradition of community-based education and training.
   1. Social work education–Fieldwork. 2. Social work education–Fieldwork–Australia.
   3. Community-based social services. 4. Community development.
   I. Westoby, Peter. II. Shevellar, Lynda.
   361.3'0723-dc23

Library of Congress Cataloging-in-Publication Data
Learning and mobilising for community development : a radical tradition of community-based education and training / [edited] by Peter Westoby and Lynda Shevellar.
      p. cm.
   Includes bibliographical references and index.
   ISBN 978-1-4094-4384-1 (hbk. : alk. paper)
   1. Community development. I. Westoby, Peter. II. Shevellar, Lynda.
   307.1'4–dc23

                                                              2012012816

ISBN 13: 978-1-138-27135-7 (pbk)
ISBN 13: 978-1-4094-4384-1 (hbk)

Contents

List of Figures

List of Tables

List of Abbreviations

AAEE	Australian Association of Environmental Education
ABL	Adventure-based Learning
ACPACS	Australian Centre for Peace and Conflict Studies
AIDS	Acquired Immunodeficiency Syndrome
ALARA	Action Learning Action Research Association
ANZSG	Australian and New Zealand Social Role Valorization Group
APY	Anangu Pitjantjatjara Yankunytjatjara (Central Australia)
ASPBAE	Asia-South Pacific Association for Basic and Adult Education
AusAID	The Australian Agency for International Development
BBC	Building Better Communities
BLP	Better Life Options Program
CBEM	Community-based Environmental Monitoring
CD	Community Development
CDRA	Community Development Resource Association
CEC-Phils	Center for Environmental Concerns-Philippines
CEDPA	Centre for Development and Population Activities
CORETECH	Community-based Rehabilitation Technology
CRC	Cooperative Research Centre
EDSA	Epifanio de los Santos Avenue (Manila, Philippines)
FA	Farmer Association
GDP	Gross Domestic Product
GPS	Global Positioning System
HIV	Human Immunodeficiency Virus
HIV/AIDS	Human Immunodeficiency Virus/Acquired Immunodeficiency Syndrome
ICAE	International Council of Adult Education
IDS	Institute of Development Studies
INGO	International Non-Government Organisation
ISSR	Institute for Social Science Research
KALACC	Kimberley Aboriginal Law and Cultural Centre
KAP	Knowledge, Attitude and Practices
LGBTIQ	Lesbian Gay Bisexual Transgender/Transexual Intersex Queer
MNCC	Malvatumauri National Council of Chiefs (Vanuatu)
NGDO	Non-Governmental Development Organisation
NGO	Non-Government Organisation
NILS	No-Interest Loan Scheme
OECD	Organisation for Economic Co-operation and Development

OPM-TPN	Organisasi Papua Merdeka - Tentara Pembebasan Nasional (Papuan National Liberation Army)
PIN	Planned Individual Networks
PLA	Participatory Learning and Action
PNG	Papua New Guinea
RENEW	Restoration Ecology Workshop
RMIT	Royal Melbourne Institute of Technology
SEI	Supplementary Education Initiative
SMO	Social Movement Organisation
SRV	Social Role Valorization
TAFE	Technical and Further Education
TB	Tuberculosis
tCA	The Change Agency
TEAR	Transformation, Empowerment, Advocacy, Relief
TfC	Training for Change
TWT	Third-Way Theatre
UK	United Kingdom
UN	United Nations
UNFPA	United Nations Population Fund
USA	United States of America
WWII	World War Two
YMCA	Young Men's Christian Association

Notes on Contributors

Dave Andrews along with his wife Ange, and their family, have worked as community workers with marginalised groups of people in Australia and Asia for 40 years. With their friends, they started the community organisations *Aashiana, Sahara* and *Sharan*, working with slum dwellers, sex workers, drug addicts and people with HIV/AIDS in India; and are currently a part of the Waiters Union, a community network working alongside Aborigines, refugees and people with disabilities in Australia.

Dave's academic background is in literature, psychology and history, education and community development. He is author of many books and articles, including *Plan Be* (2011), *Living Community* (2007), *Not Religion, But Love* (2003), and *Building a Better World* (1996). He is the community empowerment officer for Transformation, Empowerment, Advocacy, Relief (TEAR) Australia, an aid and development agency; a member of Community Praxis Co-op and an elder for Servants.

Howard Buckley was born in Queensland, Australia, and for the past 20 years he has lived in Maleny, South East Queensland with his partner and children. Howard is actively involved in community work in his local town and has played a key role in establishing the local neighbourhood centre. Howard is currently manager of a youth service on the outskirts of Brisbane, Queensland while also being actively involved in Community Praxis Co-op providing consultancy in community development training and project work in the community sector. Prior to this, he spent six years as a social planner with local government and 15 years in a variety of human service roles in the community sector.

David Denborough is a community practitioner, teacher, writer, editor and song-writer for Dulwich Centre Foundation. David's recent community work and teaching assignments have taken place in Haiti, Bosnia, Rwanda, Uganda, Palestine, Brazil, USA, Hong Kong, Canada, Chile, Argentina, Russia, Israel and a range of Australian Aboriginal communities. He is the developer or co-developer of narrative methodologies such as the Tree of Life, Team of Life and Kite of Life that are now being engaged with in a wide a range of countries. He is the author and/or editor of various books including: *Collective Narrative Practice: Responding to Individuals, Groups and Communities Who Have Experienced Trauma* (2011); *Strengthening Resistance: The Use of Narrative Practices in Working with Genocide Survivors* (2008); *Trauma: Narrative Responses to*

Traumatic Experience (2006); and *Beyond the Prison: Gathering Dreams of Freedom* (1996).

Pru Gell is a facilitator and social movement educator who works to support strategic campaign planning, coalition building and policy development. She works alongside a range of communities in urban environments and in remote Indigenous communities in Australia. Pru is passionate about working with people who want to achieve social change and facilitating strategic planning processes to support their goal. She lives in *Mparntwe* (Alice Springs) in the Australian desert on *Arrente* people's country. Indigenous peoples' rights are at the heart of her work. She is compelled to be involved in meaningful dialogue on ways forward between Indigenous peoples and others in Australia, and to explore what 'working together' really means in practice. Pru believes that story is a key ingredient in social change work.

Jose Roberto Guevara is a passionate, popular environmental educator who is committed to participatory, creative and experiential learning methodologies within the context of sustainability. He is the President of the Asia-South Pacific Association for Basic and Adult Education (ASPBAE), a network of more than 200 NGOs committed to a rights-based approach to adult learning in the region, and the Vice-President (Asia-Pacific) of the International Council of Adult Education (ICAE). Robbie is currently a Senior Lecturer in International Development at the School of Global, Urban and Social Studies at RMIT University, Social Science and Planning at RMIT University in Melbourne, Australia. His research and writing have focused on community environmental education and more recently he has branched out to examine the nature of learning partnerships for sustainability and global citizenship. He is a member of the Australian Association of Environmental Education (AAEE) and the Action Learning Action Research Association (ALARA). Robbie calls both Melbourne and Manila home.

Nicholas Haines is a community development worker whose journey in development practice began in southern India. In a village near Kanchipuram, Tamil Nadu he worked as an English tutor with a non-profit organisation that provides an academic education while preparing children for a career in *Kattaikkuttu*, a popular musical theatre of the rural poor in northern Tamil Nadu. His role was to design and facilitate English workshops that harnessed the students' passion for creative expression. After completing a Master of Development Practice at The University of Queensland in Brisbane, Australia, he headed to Cambodia to start his current job as a community development advisor at Srer Khmer, a Cambodian rural livelihoods non-government organisation (NGO). Nicholas grew up in Gympie, a small town in South East Queensland that his father describes fondly as 'the destination to which all roads lead' and 'the centre of the universe'. He loves walking through the forests and along the beaches of his home state and is hopelessly addicted to American politics.

Holly Hammond has been facilitating groups since she first became politically active at high school in the early 1990s. She has experience of activism in a number of social movements, including youth rights, women's liberation, sex industry law reform, labour rights, peace and environmentalism. She has been employed in a diverse range of community-based organisations in advocacy, publications, organising, policy, management and community development roles. In recent years she has worked as an activist educator with the Change Agency and now directs Plan to Win, a community project to assist individuals, groups and campaigns to develop the skills and clarity required to win change in the world. Holly also convenes the Melbourne Campaigners' Network to foster learning and reflection, cross-movement collaboration, and activist community.

Sam La Rocca co-founder of the Change Agency is an activist educator, organiser and researcher. Since the early 1990s, Sam has worked with a range of organisations in Australia and overseas on environmental justice and community development projects. With a love for community organising, Sam currently works with the first Greens Member of Parliament elected to the Australian federal lower house in a general election. He has also worked with Friends of the Earth International to strengthen capacity in the Asia-Pacific region for economic justice, taken direct action on climate change, strategised with East African queers, worked in solidarity with Pacific peace activists and facilitated alliances between Traditional Owners and environmental groups in Australia. Sam has a degree in environmental science and politics and was awarded first-class honours for his work understanding the factors that influence participation in grassroots social movements.

Kathy Landvogt works as a social policy researcher in Good Shepherd Youth & Family Service where she is engaged in action research, policy research and system advocacy. Currently, her research interests address issues of poverty, educational inequity, service networks and violence against women. Kathy is a social worker with experience in service delivery, management, and evaluation in both government and community-based organisations. She has also been an educator in welfare and social work, and in community and adult education. Kathy's work is founded on feminist frameworks and her PhD in social work explored active citizenship and Freirean consciousness-raising in community-based women's 'learning and support' groups.

Gregory Mackay is Director of a centre focusing on social justice advocacy, research and education in a large health and community services organisation. His academic background is in studying psychology and management, however, his key influences come from study related to the marginalisation and oppression of devalued citizen groups including those from the Peace Studies tradition. Gregory's engagement and application of community development practice has taken place within community and government ranging across management, family services, employment, accommodation, advocacy, aged care and service development.

Gregory acknowledges and pays respect to the Traditional Aboriginal Owners of the land he lives on in Brisbane, Australia.

Jason MacLeod is an activist, community development worker, educator, and researcher who has been working with local communities and social and environmental justice movements in Australia and the Asia-Pacific region since 1991. The context of this work varies, and includes conflict settings, international and local NGOs, local government, community-based organisations, and neighbourhoods and villages; although most of his work is with grassroots communities and people working for social change. He teaches civil resistance at The University of Queensland, coordinates an activist education programme in the Pacific, and is a training associate with the Change Agency. Jason is married with children, wrestles with his Quaker faith, lives in a cohousing settlement and currently has aspirations to raise chickens. Whenever possible he enjoys a long walk in wilderness country or riding a perfect pitching wave. He lives on *Jaggera* land in Brisbane, Australia.

Rennie Morello is a radical philosopher focused on the intersections between culture, spirituality, social justice and social movements. Rennie is greatly influenced by his Italian communist parents, an anthropologist and theologian who brought him to the Pacific as a young child. This is where he learned the power and history of indigenous resistance and developed a connection with Melanesian and Polynesian cultures. Rennie has a deep commitment to self-determination on multiple levels and has contributed to campaigns as an activist and educator for Aboriginal and Torres Strait Islander rights in Australia, for Romani peoples in Europe, and Ladyboys in South East Asia. In his spare time Rennie grows fresh herbs and heirloom tomatoes to make food which makes the heart sing.

David Palmer teaches in the Community Development programme at Murdoch University in Perth, Western Australia. He also spends a fair bit of time in remote Australia, looking for examples of projects that are having a positive impact on Indigenous people's lives. David's work has taken him to the southwest of Western Australia, the Kimberley, the Pilbara, the *Anangu Pitjantjatjara Yankunytjatjara* (APY) Lands in Central Australia, Alice Springs town camps and the northwest of Tasmania. He has come to the conclusion that the use of arts, performance, music, dance and film is often what makes a difference. This is because to work successfully with complex communities you need to be artful, use a repertoire of creative methods and learn to improvise. Dave often gets to travel with his partner and two gorgeous boys, lugging around swags, books, cameras, a MacBook Pro, a diabolo and a poi.

Alex Rayfield is a journalist and civil resistance educator working in the Asia-Pacific Region. Growing up as a white Australian of English, Scottish and Polish descent, Alex spent numerous years in Latin America where she worked as a newspaper editor in Chile covering popular resistance movements across Latin America. She now combines training and teaching with regular reportage of the West Papuan struggle for independence. Alex cut her popular education teeth working in solidarity with the Landless Peasants Movement in Brazil, the East Timorese struggle for independence and with environmental and Aboriginal alliances in Australia. Alex is influenced by anarchist politics that have been tempered by feminism, nonviolent action and grounded in messy experiments with solidarity. Alex is halfway through her goal of climbing the world's seven highest mountains and is currently finishing a book on indigenous civil resistance struggles.

Jane Sherwin is a Queensland-based consultant who has been involved in the lives of people who are marginalised since the late 1970s. She is a scholar-practitioner and is committed to working at a grassroots level towards a system of responsive services and supports. Jane works with groups and organisations on matters to do with values, quality, and leadership development. She has been involved in social change efforts since the early 1990s, using organisational development, systems change, training and writing as key strategies.

Lynda Shevellar is a lecturer in the Community Development Unit within the School of Social Work and Human Services at The University of Queensland, Australia. Lynda's work focuses upon the dynamics of personal, organisational and social change. She is a part of the non-profit Community Praxis Co-op, as well as a local mental health network. Lynda is influenced by 20 years of experience and study in community development, the disability sector, education, and psychology. Some of her recent work has focused upon the experience of community development workers within bureaucracy, transformative learning practice within the teaching of community development, and support for people with disabilities and mental health challenges to develop a deeper sense of community belonging. Lynda was born and bred in beautiful Byron Bay, Australia and is unable to account for her inability to tan or surf.

Sipho Sokhela is currently the National General Secretary of the South African National Council of Young Men's Christian Association (YMCA). In that role he oversees the work of 27 local associations engaged with over two thousand young people. Prior to this he was the Chief Executive Officer of the KwaZulu-Natal Council of Churches, an ecumenical agency mobilising active involvement of the church on poverty eradication and economic justice, democracy development initiatives, HIV/AIDS initiatives and peace-building. When not working Sipho loves listening to jazz, teaching young people music, playing tennis, watching soccer and movies, and being with his family nearby Durban.

Polly O. Walker has several areas of expertise including cross cultural conflict transformation, Indigenous peacemaking/conflict management, and performance peace-building. She has worked in conflict transformation research, practice and education for 15 years at The University of Queensland in the Aboriginal and Torres Strait Islander Studies Unit and The Australian Centre for Peace and Conflict Studies. Polly currently is currently Assistant Professor of Peace and Conflict Studies at Juniata College in Pennsylvania. Her academic background is in education and conflict transformation.

Peter Westoby originally hails from the UK but now loves living in Highgate Hill, Brisbane, Australia. He is currently a senior lecturer in Community Development within the School of Social Work and Human Services at The University of Queensland, Australia and a Research Fellow with the Centre for Development Support, University of Free State, South Africa. He is also a Director/consultant with the non-profit Community Praxis Co-op. Peter's experience includes over 20 years of development practice work in South Africa, PNG, the Philippines, Vanuatu and Australia. He is also the author of several books including *Dialogical Community Development* (2009) and *The Sociality of Refugee Healing* (2009). In his spare time Peter also loves drinking good coffee, hanging out in his local book shop Avid Reader, travelling to remote parts of the planet and bush walking.

James Whelan lives in Newcastle, Australia in the *Worimi* nation. His commitment to community action for social and environmental justice has drawn him to work in the community sector, and in research and higher education. As a community educator and activist, James has worked with non-government and grassroots community and environment groups. As a researcher and lecturer, James has worked with several Australian universities. He was theme leader for the Coastal Cooperative Research Centre's Citizen Science research programme, has published widely on participatory democracy and social movements and has spoken at national and international conferences. James' community and academic worlds merge in his work as director of the Change Agency, a non-profit organisation which provides education, training, facilitation and action research support for social change groups throughout Australia and the Pacific.

Foreword

This collection could scarcely be more relevant for those concerned with community development in the context of wider agendas for equalities and social justice. As engaged scholars, the editors have provided a critical framework within which to explore a range of experiences of community-based education and training, unpacking the concepts and retrieving their progressive potential. The collection starts by emphasising the values and traditions of community learning and mobilisation, rooted in mutuality, reciprocity and dialogue. Although the editors emphasise mutuality and dialogue, they are also clear about the importance of the educator's role. They point, for instance, to the example of Rosa Parks, the black woman who played such a key role in struggles for civil rights in the USA. Far from being a spontaneous act, Rosa Parks' courageous defiance of the segregation laws which sparked off the bus boycott, at the beginning of the Civil Rights Movement, was the conscious decision of a committed activist who had benefited from progressive learning at the Highlander Center in Tennessee, USA.

Having set out the case for the educator's importance, the editors unpack and reclaim the radical traditions of community-based education and training, emphasising the importance of reflexively locating practice within these different traditions. While the experiences and the narratives that form the basis for these reflections from practice have been rooted in Australia, the Balkans, South East Asia, the Pacific and South Africa, the underlying issues and dilemmas resonate so much more widely. This is why the book will make an important contribution more generally. This is over and above its contribution, providing insights into learning and mobilising for community development in diverse settings including Vanuatu, West Papua and the Philippines, settings that have been less familiar for many readers.

Learning to take part in civil society has emerged as a highly topical policy commitment in the current context, in Britain, as in other places too. The UK Coalition Government's Big Society programme to train 500 senior community organisers and 4, 500 mid-level community organisers has been described by Locality, the Third Sector organisation delivering the programme, as a 'once-in-a-generation opportunity to engage vast numbers of people in positive community-led action' (Locality, 2010). Drawing upon the learning approaches developed by both Paulo Freire and Saul Alinsky, the programme aims to provide the means for people – 'who are most excluded from the inner circles of power and privilege – to combine and be counted, to discover their ability to identify those changes which will mean most to them and, on their own terms, take action to tackle vested interests' realising the goal of the Big Society as a society 'where no-one is made to feel small' (Locality 2010). Locality's strategy for delivering the Coalition Government's Community Organisers programme started by recognising the value of a Freirean-based community education model. But Freirean learning methods needed to be supplemented with an organising approach, with a hard edge of political engagement, if local people were to be effectively heard by the powerful, Locality argued (Locality, 2010).

This links directly into the theoretical debates that underpin this collection. How far though might a community organising approach be more effective in these practical terms, delivering more immediate impacts in terms of issues, such as planning and service delivery? And how far might such an approach be sustainable in the current context, especially at a time when the fundamental fabric of social welfare provision in Britain is being challenged (Taylor-Gooby and Stoker, 2011)? Critics of the Big Society have pointed to the contradictions inherent in inviting the Third Sector to play an increasingly prominent role against this background of public expenditure cuts – not only to public sector organisations and services but also to voluntary and community sector organisations and infrastructure alike. Although these contradictions are far from being entirely new, public sector retrenchment is arguably on a different scale altogether, in the current policy context, posing challenges of a new order (Taylor-Gooby and Stoker, 2011). How far then might the inclusion of an Alinsky style approach resolve some of the limitations that Locality identified as inherent in previous initiatives?

The Introduction and first chapters of this collection are particularly valuable in addressing these questions, unpacking the concepts and differing approaches, including differing approaches to learning and differing approaches to community development more generally. These chapters include critical examinations of the approaches developed by both Paulo Freire and Saul Alinsky. There are similarities, but there are also significant differences between Freirean based models and Alinsky based models, although both approaches have been interpreted in varying ways, in practice. Such differences of definition, interpretation and strategy are central to the issues that are explored by the editors, setting the scene for the development of the types of critical understanding needed to address these questions reflectively.

My own view is that the following passage is also helpful. In conversation with Paulo Freire, Myles Horton of the Highlander Research and Education Center in Tennessee explained that, although he had been a staunch supporter of Saul Alinsky – and vice versa, 'we differed and we recognized the difference. We had no problem about it, and we tried to explain to people that there was a difference' (Bell et al. 1990: 115). Horton went on to argue that, 'basically it's [that is, education at the Highlander Center] not technical training. We're not in the technical business. We emphasize ways you analyse and perform and relate to people, but that's what I call education not organizing' (Bell et al. 1990: 116). The analysis of the underlying causes of social problems and social injustices was central to this approach – education as the basis for long term strategies for social justice. Alinsky's approach, in contrast, was perceived as being centrally concerned with mobilising to attain achievable targets in the here and now. The question facing the Community Organisers programme in England, then, may be how to define and combine the strengths of both approaches and how to apply these in practice, organising to achieve practical goals, whilst enabling communities to develop longer term strategies for social change.

This would seem to have particular relevance, in view of the fundamental challenges to the Welfare State that are being posed at a time when poverty in Britain is predicted to rise, and public spending to be cut back to a lower proportion of GDP than public spending in the USA by 2013 (Taylor-Gooby and Stoker, 2011). Attempts to further roll back the Welfare State risk re-enforcing the view that the responsibility for responding to increasing social needs and widening social inequalities should lie with civil society, in general, and with active citizens more specifically. This could indeed be more oppressive rather than more empowering as an outcome, both for individuals and for communities, posing major dilemmas for those engaged in working with communities.

This collection has particular relevance then, for those engaged in promoting learning and mobilising for community development in the current context. The book's final chapter draws upon the learning from the previous chapters, with their 12 different stories, constructing a seven dimensional framework for guiding practice for community development practitioners. This could provide valuable insights for those concerned with providing community-based learning as part of wider strategies, working towards social justice and equalities agendas for the future.

Marjorie Mayo
July 2012

References

Bell, B., Gaventa, J. and Peters, J. eds, 1990. *We Make the Road by Walking: Conversations on Education and Social Change, Myles Horton and Paulo Freire*. Philadelphia: Temple University Press.

Locality, 2010, *Tender to Provide a National Partner for the Community Organisers Programme* [Online: Locality]. Available at: www.locality.org.uk/wp-content/uploads/Locality-CO-web-25052011.pdf [accessed: 5 December 2011].

Taylor-Gooby, P. and Stoker, G., 2011, 'The Coalition programme: A new vision for Britain or politics as usual?' *The Political Quarterly*, 82(1), 4–15.

Acknowledgements

As a *collective of author-activists* who have worked around the globe, we share the privilege of being exposed to some of the most inspiring community-based trainers and educators, the luxury of reading the works of other author-activists, and, perhaps most significantly, the honour of standing alongside communities in their struggle for transformation and justice. This is our context for learning, therefore, to try and single out people to acknowledge formally is an almost impossible task. So we simply offer our thanks to those who continue to touch our lives, both present and past.

However, as *editors* we would like to express our gratitude to the chapter authors: Dave Andrews, Howard Buckley, David Denborough, Pru Gell, Jose Roberto Guevara, Nicholas Haines, Holly Hammond, Sam La Rocca, Kathy Landvogt, Gregory Mackay, Jason MacLeod, Rennie Morello, David Palmer, Alex Rayfield, Jane Sherwin, Sipho Sokhela, Polly Walker and James Whelan. Their contributions, as grounded stories of practice, are the soul of the book. We are of course grateful to all those people who made the stories the above authors told possible. Also, our heartfelt thanks to Marjorie Mayo for taking the time to read the manuscript and pen the Foreword.

Of course the editorial process is a lengthy one – and we are truly grateful for the work of Meredith Connor who worked carefully and diligently through the whole text to massage sentences, pick up grammatical mistakes and review for references.

We would also like to acknowledge the support our efforts have received from the institutions we work within, both The University of Queensland, Australia, and also the Free State University, South Africa.

Finally, we would like to thank our partners – Larah and Robert – for without their patience, care and love, such writing would not be possible.

Peter Westoby and Lynda Shevellar
July 2012

Introduction

Peter Westoby and Lynda Shevellar

'Could you provide us with some training…'
'As a community group we need some training in…'

As engaged scholars in the field of community development, we regularly find ourselves in conversations that begin with these phrases. We are approached to 'provide training' to assist groups of people and their organisations to engage with the ideas and practices of community development. As practitioners who are also members of a community workers co-operative, we are often invited to work with groups of residents who want us to accompany them in learning about how to make their neighbourhoods a better place for themselves and those who are marginalised.

Almost any community worker will have had similar requests and invitations. Education and training processes are integral elements of much community development work.

This book is our attempt to make sense of such community-based education and training work. However, in this attempt we also recognise the paradox that is created by a call for expertise in developmental work and all that this implies. The critiques of education and development as subjugating technologies are well known (Gareau 2003, Chege 2009, Redfern 2009). At the same time, located within the Australian Higher Education system, we find ourselves both colluding with and actively resisting the colonising practices of our formal education system.

Our analysis emerges from our wrestling with these tensions. Do we discard the language of education and training because it has been captured by conventional development paradigm assumptions? How could we reclaim the language and reorient the practice? How might we enter into dialogue about how community-based education and training is conceptualised, mandated, planned, designed, and evaluated? How do we support the interplay between group/collective learning and action within community development theory and practice?

In engaging with such tensions we explore a body of knowledge, theory and practice that we think of as community-based education and training. This book has at its core two main arguments: firstly, following on from our opening comments, we are concerned with an increasingly instrumental approach to community development whereby 'experts' are seen to know best, thereby undermining a genuine process of groups of people learning together. As a counterpoint to this, the *social learning* approach (Campfens 1997) supports the process of collectives of people learning together, generating an analysis together, and choosing and implementing collective actions together. Some of the more contemporary discourses around such practices would include participatory learning and action (Pretty et al. 1995, Chambers 2007), horizontal learning (CDRA 2004–2005) and capacity building (Oswald and Clarke 2010, Ubels, Acquaye-Baddoo and Fowler 2010); although they can just as easily be captured by an instrumental ethos (Kenny and Clarke 2010).

Secondly, in this book we assert that it is not enough to learn and then wish for social change: it is not enough to 'hope'. Drawing upon the *social mobilisation* approach (Campfens 1997), we seek community development that also builds collective organisational strength. Some of the contemporary thinking here draws on strengths and assets-based (Mathie and Cunningham 2008) and rights-based (Ife 2010) approaches to community development. There is the need to 'confront' power with power, so to speak, within organisational forms. The idea of social mobilisation frames community development as a method for those who are marginalised to organise together and act collectively through these structures, to challenge the way the systemically powerful wish to make decisions, allocate resources and control agendas.

This book therefore demonstrates the importance and the possibilities of community-based education and training in creating social change. However, its significance lies beyond this. Through practitioner stories, in Parts II and III, we analyse the practices and applications, the challenges, the limitations and even the failings of community-based education and training approaches. Our intention is to draw upon stories to provide a highly accessible means of thinking about community-based education and training that goes beyond the usual step-by-step approaches to development, and instead explores the tensions and conflicts that accompany this complex work.

Three wonderful stories of community-based education and training that have inspired our social imagination illustrate the significance of linking community-based education and training to learning and mobilising traditions of community development. The first story that captivates us is that of Rosa Parks 'triggering' the civil rights movement within the USA. For many years, both of us had heard this story through the lens of the 'lone hero'. Here was a weary African American who simply got to the point of saying 'enough' and refusing to move on the bus for a white passenger when asked. But over time, we learnt of the extraordinary deliberation and solidarity infused in this act. Rosa Parks, along with so many other African American community members and emerging leaders had already participated in the community-based training programme initiated by the Highlander Folk Institute led by Myles Horton and his colleagues. She was ready for change as were the Highlander trained African American leaders who then mobilised people into action. The role of long-term community-based education and training – in this case training in analysis, nonviolence and collective action – cannot be underestimated.

The second story that has intrigued us is the account of community-based nonviolence training that had gone on for many years prior to the Philippines EDSA (Epifanio de los Santos Avenue) People Power Revolution of 1986. At this time, one of the editors, Peter, had just started his journey in undergraduate education and had been captivated by this 'EDSA Revolution'. In his youthful naivety, he was amazed by the seemingly spontaneous combustion of people into disciplined direct action demanding justice and human rights. Such imagination inspired his hopes that people around the world might one day 'wake-up' to the social forces of domination and exploitation at work within their lives and the world and resist. However, in visiting the Philippines he learnt of the significant preparation that had gone into laying the foundation for such action. That preparation consisted of many learning groups led by progressive elements within the Catholic Church (influenced deeply by liberation theology) and non-government organisations (NGOs) using popular education and nonviolence training. The kind of transformative action that we often hope for does not spontaneously occur. It requires painstaking groundwork in community-based education and training to assist people to understand their world and gather the collective courage required to act against forces of domination.

The third and final story for this Introduction is that of Father Arizmendi's study circles within the initial years of forming the Mondragón co-operative movement. As members of an Australian workers co-operative, and therefore as people intrigued by the complexities – both delightful and at times incredibly difficult – of co-operating, we have often wondered how to build a more ethically-focused and community-oriented economy. The Mondragón co-operative movement of the Basque region of Spain has always been an inspiration to co-operators around the world. Again, the unseen work is time invested by Father Arizmendi. He started his community work in the region in 1941, yet only established the first co-operative in 1956. Those 15 in-between years were spent initiating many community ventures, but a key was conducting more than two thousand study circles on social, humanist and religious topics (Whyte and Whyte 1988, 1991: 29–32). It was in the context of such study circles that the Basques learnt how to [re]create themselves as associational people able to co-operate in economic affairs.

Such stories illustrate the importance of community-based education and training within community development work. The first two stories focus on learning that leads to mobilisation; both in forms of civic-led action that confronts political power. The last story focuses on learning that leads to economic action through the formation of co-operative organisations.

We tell these three stories because they have been personally inspiring to us, and because they provide a glimpse into history, albeit still running its course: the race struggles of the USA; the people's struggles against systemic power within the Philippines; and the Mondragón attempt to re-imagine and re-organise economic relations. Community-based education and training has such a rich and clearly radical history. It is this kind of history, and the tradition it represents, that the collective of writers here would like to revitalise.

However, in uplifting community-based education and training, and praising its potential, we are also conscious there are places of uncertainty and contestation beneath our seemingly confident narrative. This contested territory is illuminated by sharing the key debates that have taken place among the collective of authors in this book. These debates have focused upon the nature of 'education' and 'training', the idea of a 'radical' orientation and the problem of authority. As editors, to this list we would add the challenges of authorship and 'voice'. Each of these debates are now discussed.

The most vigorous author debate focused on community-based *education* and community-based *training*, that is, whether this is about education or training within community settings. Some of the debate has emerged because of divergent 'traditions' of practice that writers come from. Some of the writers come from activist traditions, others from community building and community development; a few are deeply influenced by feminist literature; and others by conflict transformation. Each tradition, underpinned by different disciplines, uses language in different ways. For those within a community building tradition the word 'training' holds the combination of learning and action (see for example Hope and Timmel 1984). For some others within the collective, training is a heavily loaded word, indicative of professionalisation and job preparedness skills orientation. This is particularly the case in Part II of the book and stories intersecting with the Australian training system, given its present focus on competency-based training. This is a highly regulated, instrumental, professionalised and industry-oriented training system rarely, if ever, critical of contemporary social, economic, cultural or political trajectories.

To engage with this tension as editors we simply mined our own autobiographical experience in education and training. For both of us, many experiences of education were domesticating; school was geared towards being job-ready, defined by a pre-determined curriculum that often felt removed from our learning interests. However, over the years we have both discovered more progressive and liberating traditions of education. Thus we started to ask ourselves, 'Are there more radical or liberating traditions of training as well?' And of course there are. The three stories told above provide a glimpse of such a tradition.

As such, we do not want to perpetuate the binary of progressive education and conservative training – although we do acknowledge nuances in meaning. From our perspective, it is useful to think of community-based *education* as signifying a process that is about learning for the purposes of 'increasing awareness' or 'acquiring new knowledge or skills', whereas community-based *training* signifies a movement towards action emergent from a participatory and democratic process among a group of people. There is a subtle shift when we consider the difference between the two words education and training. As a reader if you cannot quite appreciate the difference, consider if someone came up to you and offered a class to your teenage daughter on 'sex education'. Now consider if the offer was for 'sex training'! Despite this distinction, we argue that both education and training discourses and practices can be domesticating or they can be liberating. Hence, we have decided to work with both terms.

The second key debate concerns the use of the term 'radical'. One of our ambitions is to contribute to the revitalisation of community-based education and training practice as radical practice – hence the sub-title of the book *A Radical Tradition of Community-based Education and Training*. This rich practice tradition has been recently articulated by Stephen Brookfield and John Holst in their book *Radicalizing Learning* (2010). It is further represented by powerful practical publications, such as Anne Hope and Sally Timmel's *Training for Transformation: A Handbook for Community Workers* (Volumes I–IV) first published in 1984, drawing on Paulo Freire's philosophy of learning, and also by T. R. Batten's early classic *Training for Community Development: A Critical Study of Method* (1962).

In drawing on the idea of 'radical' we need to be clear. We adopt the spirit of the word used by Brookfield and Holst (2010: 3) who see being radical 'as getting to the roots of something to discover the essence'. In this sense, community-based education and training has 'roots' that are linked to processes whereby groups of people come together in a process of social learning for the purposes of collective action. Such action, for us, is understood as social mobilisation. It is not about domesticating education and training where people are prepared for jobs within the capitalist mainstream. Rather it is radical action aimed at creating cooperative power and challenging existing power.

However, unlike Brookfield and Holst, we do not believe this radical action *necessarily* implies pathways to socialism. For us, the processes of social learning and social mobilisation that take place within community-based education and training are guided by the people. The people determine the pathways. Educators or trainers can engage in processes of instruction, facilitation and even provocation: challenging beliefs, assumptions, and chosen actions. Ultimately, it is the participants in a group who determine actions and pathways as they learn collectively and mobilise themselves. Those of us laying claim to using community-based education and training as radicals would ideally see such learning and mobilising challenge abuses of power as expressed through structures of patriarchy, racism, colonialism and class relations. However, our commitment to core community development principles and orthodoxies would not enable us to manipulate groups ideologically. The community-based education and training space is a dialogical space, one in which trainers can bring their perspectives, their ideas; however, they cannot afford to exert ideological control. The roots of community development practice are held firmly in its 'good memes' (Chambers 2005: 152) such as: 'hold your agenda lightly', 'hand over the pen', 'ask them', 'sit down, listen and learn', 'start with the people', 'ask questions and invite questions'. Thus there is faith that a dialogical space will lead to group wisdom, analysis and agreed upon actions.

The third tension raised in the development of this book challenges the link between education/training and 'development experts'. Conventional development paradigms are founded on ideas and practices of 'transfer' where transfer signifies the movement of either technology or expertise from 'developed' to 'undeveloped' countries/contexts. In this space external experts usually educate or train 'the locals'. Within this paradigm education and training becomes a social technology, reinforcing the problematic assumptions and practices of the conventional development paradigm. It should also be noted that even more contemporary language/concepts – such as capacity building – can suffer the same fate, with the assumption being that people of the North capacitate people of the South (see the work of Linda Tuhiwai Smith 1999). It is pertinent that all three of the stories at the start of this Introduction reflect journeys of education and training initiated from within cultural contexts, albeit a deeper examination of the stories illuminates the useful role of outsiders.

We are sensitive to the damage that has occurred because of the interventions of well-intentioned 'experts' throughout history. Yet, at the same time, we wish to problematise the binary of expert and novice. In the community-based education and training context learning occurs as a dynamic through relationship – not as a product through transmission. This is not to suggest the absence of power dynamics, but rather that dynamics are negotiated rather than imposed, and as our final chapter explores, context is all-important. As trainers we often work alongside local trainers, utilising educational opportunities as vehicles for local skill building. Many of the authors have lived, as well as worked in the communities they discuss here. Others are mindful of their ongoing outsider status despite years of experience, and bearing witness to a community's struggles. As educators/trainers entering learning spaces effectively means we need to work with humility and to embrace our own ongoing learner status. Thus, we imagine learning not as an expert-trainer transaction, but as a dynamic of mutual transformation.

Accompanying the issue of expertise is the fourth debate that has perhaps been most evident to us as editors of this collection, the issue of voice. While the voices of training participants are woven into these stories they do not appear as co-authors. Authors include academics and researchers, as well as local activists and change agents. In this way, the book provides a space for interplay between theory and practice, which in turn widens the potential audience and its application. At the same time, we recognise the limitations of this endeavour. As illustrated in the next section, the author-practitioners were chosen for their depth of experience, a breadth of practice context, clarity about their approach and recognition of the integrity of their work, not merely their institutional affiliation or any attempt at representativeness.

With this in mind, we now turn to an overview of the book.

Organisation of Book and Overview of the Chapters

The book is organised in four parts. Part I outlines the key elements that underpin effective community-based education and training. It then locates community-based education and training within a broader pedagogical project, by tracing the tradition of transformative learning and education. This part of the book consists of the two opening chapters that are theory oriented. They should provide the reader with some touchstones when reading the stories of Parts II and III. Chapter 1 considers community-based education and training conceptually, as part of community development theory and practice. It particularly focuses on our key perspectives for re-thinking community-based education and training. This is achieved by considering our understanding of community as dialogue versus collectivity, the 'base' of community-based types of knowledge within the practice, and finally different traditions of community development that underpin the work.

Chapter 2 traces the traditions of thought that underpin community-based education and training, focusing on adult and transformative learning, as well as popular education. The aim of this chapter is to provide a comprehensive understanding of the ideas, key authors and texts that inform the practice.

Parts II and III focus on stories and practice, distilling the application of theory and frameworks in particular settings. Part II consists of six stories of Australian practice in diverse contexts from The Kimberley through to inner city Melbourne.

Chapter 3, written by David Palmer provides an account of attempts by Indigenous communities to support their young people in the Kimberley area of Western Australia. It offers a story of Elders who are reigniting old systems of education. The chapter describes how desert people think about, and carry out what we often call 'education and training'. In particular, it explores the important part that relationships (skin), place (country) and narrative (story) play in knowledge transfer across generations. In this way, the chapter provides an example of how traditional law and cultural practices have been used to influence the solutions a community seeks.

Within Chapter 4, Kathy Landvogt tells the story of the innovative use of community-based education to achieve research and policy advocacy goals in the context of an Australian community service organisation. The organisation's theatre training project tapped the voices of those most adversely affected by the 'money system' and resulted in engaging a group of women in a 'Theatre of the Oppressed' dialogic learning process. As well as discussing the thinking and the practices that underpinned the project, this chapter will outline some of the difficulties and benefits of using theatre education for research and advocacy purposes.

James Whelan and his colleagues reflect on their 'Strategising for Change' action research project in Chapter 5. The project, which began in 2003, has resulted in strategy workshops, the mentoring of campaigners and the development of a suite of resources to assist with analysis and strategic planning. In the process, the authors learnt not only about campaign strategy, but also about political education and 'conscientisation'.

In Chapter 6 Lynda Shevellar, Jane Sherwin and Gregory Mackay argue that, although traditional education approaches have been effective in raising consciousness, and assisting people to develop an understanding of the main issues affecting people with disabilities, the absence of community-based education and training has resulted in a lack of action in recent years. Drawing on a case study of a community-based organisation, they consider what community-based training and education approaches might offer the disability sector, and use these experiences to imagine a movement from heightened consciousness to a commitment to action.

Howard Buckley, in Chapter 7, tells the story of how one local government authority tried to respond to the question of 'Where is community and how do you build it?' in the context of rapid population growth and urban development. As this chapter details, the result was Building Better Communities (BBC): a reflective journey of self-development in relationship with others that led to skills development and collaborative action.

In Chapter 8 Dave Andrews, explores the dynamics of *In Situ* Community Work Training currently delivered through an inner city intentional-community network known as the Waiters Union, located in West End, Brisbane. This network seeks to develop the kind of community that is inclusive of, and committed to, marginalised and disadvantaged groups people in the local neighbourhood.

Part III moves to a global perspective with stories from Europe to the Pacific. Polly Walker explores training conducted within the Vanuatu *Kastom* governance project, a partnership between the Malvatumauri National Council of Chiefs (MNCC), The Australian Centre for Peace and Conflict Studies (ACPACS) and the Australian Agency for International Development (AusAID). A central aspect of the partnership is the facilitation of elicitive, dialogical workshops, called *storians*, designed to draw on Ni-Vanuatu values, frameworks and processes while integrating new skills that serve to strengthen Ni-Vanuatu governance.

In Chapter 10, Nicholas Haines tackles the challenge of cultural change in assisting trainers to move from a transfer mode of training and education to a more inclusive and learner focused interaction. Through his discussion of famer training in Cambodia, he articulates a participatory learning approach. His thoughtful account reflects on changes in the learning experience not only with the target group of farmers, but perhaps more significantly, changes among his colleague-trainers/educators and himself.

David Denborough then explores the question of how training programmes can contribute to the 'invention of unity in diversity'. He draws on a story of how collective narrative practices, which were the focus of the training, were engaged with in order to build peace within Srebrenica. Chapter 11 also introduces a range of collective narrative practices and describes how these are relevant to community development, while also examining the interface of pedagogy, peace-building and community development.

Chapter 12 explores the work of the Freedom Project, a project designed to transform vertical conflict and support democratic transitions in West Papua through promoting and strengthening civil resistance. Alex Rayfield and Rennie Morello argue that there is a need for educators to stand with the oppressed and work hand in hand for liberation. The problem is that to do that, is to *bikin kacau* – to stir up trouble for yourself, your life and for others – as well as, laying some foundations for a more sustainable and just peace. This chapter holds out the belief in the need to practice liberatory education and tangible solidarity with people actively engaged in political struggle.

In Chapter 13, Jose Roberto Guevara reflects on the development of a grassroots environmental education curriculum by the Center for Environmental Concerns-Philippines (CEC-Phils) – an environmental NGO that works in conjunction with educators from NGOs and sectoral organisations of women, farmers, fisherfolk, urban poor and indigenous peoples. The chapter will look at two levels of contextualisation and argue that it was a sharper political-ecological perspective that helped develop a contexutalised curriculum.

In Chapter 14, Peter Westoby and Sipho Sokhela tell the story of the Better Life Options Program (BLP), a community-based, peer education initiative of the South African National Council of YMCAs. The programme seeks to mobilise young people in their communities around learning and action (local and national), and to address issues of reproductive health education generally and HIV specifically.

Part IV consists of the final chapter, drawing on key wisdom from the previous stories of practice, and articulating the dimensions of a proposed education and training framework. In this chapter the editors, Peter Westoby and Lynda Shevellar, posit that such a framework might well be useful for practitioners engaged in social learning and mobilisation within community settings. The purpose in doing this is twofold. Firstly, it provides a framework for practitioners who might be working intuitively, or 'flying by the seat of their pants', so to speak. For such practitioners such a framework might help in being more disciplined or conscious in the work. Secondly, for practitioners who are already working with an education and training framework, there is an invitation to initiate deeper reflection, and invite consideration of new practice wisdom.

References

Batten, T.R. 1962. *Training for Community Development: A Critical Study of Method*. London: Oxford University Press.

Brookfield, S.D. and Holst, J.D. 2010. *Radicalizing Learning: Adult Education for a Just World*. San Francisco: John Wiley.

Campfens, H. 1997. *Community Development Around the World: Practice, Theory, Research, Training*. Toronto: University of Toronto Press.

CDRA, 2004–2005. *Horizontal Learning: Engaging Freedom's Possibilities*. South Africa: Community Development Resource Association.

Chambers, R. 2005. *Ideas for Development*. London: Earthscan.

Chambers, R. 2007. From PRA to PLA to pluralism: Practice and theory. IDS Working Paper 286. Sussex: Institute of Development Studies.

Chege, M. 2009. The politics of education in Kenyan universities: A call for a paradigm shift. *African Studies Review*, 52(3), 55–71.

Gareau, M.M. 2003. Colonization within the university system, *The American Indian Quarterly, Special Issue: Native Experiences in the Ivory Tower*, 27(1–2), 196–9.

Hope, A. and Timmel, S. 1984. *Training for Transformation: A Handbook for Community Workers*. Zimbabwe: Mambo Press.

Ife, J. 2010. *Human Rights from Below: Achieving Rights Through Community Development*. Cambridge: Cambridge University Press.

Kenny, S. and Clarke, M. eds, 2010. *Challenging Capacity Building: Comparative Perspectives*. Basingstoke: Palgrave Macmillan.

Mathie, A. and Cunningham, G. eds, 2008. *From Citizens to Clients: Communities Changing the Course of Their Own Development*. Warwickshire: Intermediate Technology Publications.

Oswald, K. and Clarke, P. 2010. Reflecting collectively on capacities for change. *Institute of Development Studies Bulletin*, 41(3).

Pretty, J., Guijt, I., Thompson, J. and Scoones, I. 1995. *A Trainer's Guide for Participatory Learning and Action*. London: Sustainable Agriculture Programme, International Institute for Environment and Development.

Redfern, J. 2009. My story: Colonization, sexuality and Aboriginal youthfalse. *Our Schools, Our Selves*, 18(2), 11–16.

Smith, L. T. 1999. *Decolonizing Methodologies: Research and Indigenous Peoples*. London: Zed Books.

Ubels, J., Acquaye-Baddoo, N. and Fowler, A. (eds). 2010. *Capacity Development in Practice*. London: Earthscan.

Whyte, W.F. and Whyte, K.K. 1988. *Making Mondragón: The Growth and Dynamics of the Worker Cooperative Complex*. New York: ILR Press.

Whyte, W.F. and Whyte, K.K. 1991. *Making Mondragón: The Growth and Dynamics of the Worker Cooperative Complex*. Second Edition Revised. New York: ILR Press.

PART I
A Radical Tradition of Community-based Education and Training

Chapter 1

A Perspective on Community-based Education and Training

Peter Westoby and Lynda Shevellar

Community as Dialogue and Collectivity

Within normative community development processes people come together because they share some common concern. This 'coming together' usually emerges *organically* – people find one another within their existing networks, or it can happen *purposefully* – someone such as a community worker, leader or activist enables it to happen through networking and inviting people to come together. In this process of coming together people discover the possibilities and potentials of cooperation. People learn or realise that what they could not do or make sense of alone, they can do as a group. Within community development methodology a key part of this process is the shift from what is sometimes understood as 'I' to 'We'. It is a critical shift, a significant movement. It is the *formation* or construction of community (Brent 2009).

We use the word community here synonymously with the collective, but with a key caveat. For us, community as a collective signifies the 'in-between' space of individuality and a kind of collective 'group-think'. Therefore, we are careful in using the concept of collective taking heed of Martin Buber's (1947, 2002: 37) warning that 'Collectivity is based on an organised atrophy of personal existence ... [it] is a flight from community's testing and consecration of the person, a flight from the vital dialogic, demanding the staking of the self, which is in the heart of the world.' Community then is carefully theorised as a form of collectivity in which individuals are not collapsed into group-think; it honours the individuals, but enfolds it within a mutual process of dialogue and participation with others.

It is important to understand this 'in-between space' – between individuality and group-think – that enables groups to form and in which individuals, conscious of their mutual relationship with others, create spaces for both learning and action. For us, holding such a space requires a deep understanding of dialogue within community-based development work. Such understanding builds on two key ideas of Buber, each of which is now discussed.

I-It vs. I-Thou: Mutuality within Development Practice

At the crux of Buber's contribution to an understanding of dialogue is his seminal work *I-Thou* (1958). Our reading of this work leads to an argument that there are two key ways of experiencing the world generally and relationships specifically. The first, characterised as *I-It* is understood as an experience of object-subject. In a community-based education and training context this would occur if, for example, a government agency, social movement organisation (SMO) or a development practitioner decided that 'a community needs some training'. The community in this case is objectified – perceived as 'it': some passive 'other' that requires intervention.

In contrast, Buber discusses subject-subject relations as *I-Thou*. They are characterised as relations of mutuality, equal exchange, and connection. Within this latter kind of relationship, people or communities are referred to not as clients, customers or consumers, but as people, constituents and co-creators in a learning and action process. The emphasis is on the mutuality and reciprocity potentially embedded in all relationships. Such a shift entails developing a philosophical orientation, or more aptly, an attitude towards self and other that is characterised by a dialogical connection of mutuality and reciprocity. To imagine such relating is to imagine opportunities for re-humanising, which re-centre people as active agents making decisions, using their creativity, resources, relationship and intelligence. An *I-Thou* relationship is a space that focuses our efforts on relationship building, storytelling, deep listening and building a shared commitment to change.

The Structure of Dialogue: Building Connection and Commitment for Change

Part of the challenge of creating space for the possibility of community as dialogue, and therefore resisting group-think forms of collectivity, is to have some understanding of the structure of dialogue. Such understanding enables people to become technically adept in at least creating the conditions in which community can be fostered, and the kind of community-based education and training that we envisage can occur.

One element of the structure of Buber's dialogue has previously been interpreted and described technically in terms of first, second and third movement (Kelly and Burkett, 2008) and has been articulated and drawn here to offer directionality for community practice. As interpreted by Anthony Kelly and Sandra Sewell (1988), Buber identified three connected and enfolding 'movements' in our dialogue with others. The idea of three enfolding movements clarifies a dynamic process. For instance, 'first movement' interaction 'occurs when we present ourselves to another, or others...we say hello, say who we are and why we are there' (Kelly and Burkett 2008: 49). 'Second movement' dialogue occurs when there is a response from the other to our first movement statements (Kelly and Burkett 2008). 'Third movement' dialogue 'occurs when there is a response to the response' (Kelly and Burkett 2008: 50). It requires practitioners to be attentive to what is being said,

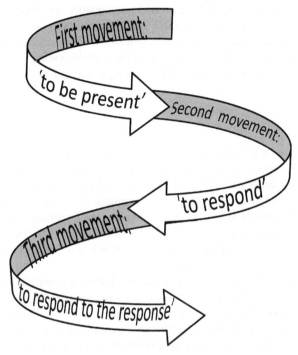

Adapted from: Kelly and Burkett 2008, Westoby and Owen 2010.

Figure 1.1   The movement structure of dialogue

to listen for and connect with what is being communicated. Genuine dialogue, in Buber's usage, necessarily goes through all three movements, folding back and forth in reciprocal fashion. Buber describes this process of establishing 'mutual' relationships as a condition of moving from 'I' (first movement) to 'You' (second movement) to 'We' (third movement) (Figure 1.1).

The challenge of understanding and applying such structure in dialogue is to be ever attentive to the perspective of people encountered. Many people remain 'stuck' in first and second movement exchanges returning constantly to their own agendas, unable to enter the other person's world. There is, therefore, minimal possibility of understanding the world of the other, of grasping their experience or perspective. Clearly, such dialogic structure is pertinent when imagining community as dialogue within education and training settings. Many such settings are structured as hierarchical institutions, or foster hierarchical dynamics that do not create spaces where people can necessarily listen deeply to one another responding to the issues of the 'other'. People, focused on their *ascribed roles* as leader, trainer, teacher, development expert and so forth, are often unable to encounter one another in *dialogical relationship* with an orientation to understanding each other's different worlds. It is our sense that some of the more contemporary thinking around participatory approaches to learning, such as articulated by Chambers (2007), and Kumar (2002) are trying to create, via participatory techniques, spaces and platforms which enable such listening and connecting. For us, Buber's ideas provide a philosophical take on how to understand what Chambers and Kumar are trying to achieve.

Community-*based*

Having discussed our understanding of community and dialogue we now turn to the notion of 'community-*based*'. In writing a book about community-based education and training we ask the question: What does it mean to be community-based? The perspective we bring is that 'community-based' signifies two key ideas. The first is that 'community-based' signifies the importance of the learning process connecting at a 'grassroots' level. The second idea is to think of 'base' in terms of 'people in place 'taking responsibility'' (Kelly and Sewell 1988: 49). Each of these ideas is now discussed in turn.

In the terms of the first idea, to undertake community-based education and training, rather than organisational-based or sector-based training, is to be involved in training that takes place *amongst* people who directly have a concern within their locality, or within their interest or identity group. In the same way that community development is different to sector development, or organisational development – in that the word 'community' signifies not only a dialogical relationship, but a connection at the grassroots within development work – so it is in education and training work. If training is conducted amongst a group of professionals working within a service delivery organisation, then it is not 'community-based' education/ training, it is professional-based or sector-based training.

The second idea signified by 'community-based' is that of thinking about base in terms of taking responsibility. We draw on a useful framework again originally articulated by Kelly and Sewell (1988: 42) as 'space, place, and base'. Within this framework *space* is understood as a geographical area in which people live or are located. Some people simply occupy space – for example, they dwell in a space, come and go to work and home, but have little connection to it. However, for some people the relationship to space shifts as they develop a sense of connection to the space, and derive a sense of belonging. The space now thought about as a *place*, rather than just space is a part of their identity (Kelly and Sewell 1988: 47). Furthermore, some people not only derive a sense of belonging from a place, but also decide to take responsibility for it. Within the framework, at this point such people have made the location their *base*. In a sense then some people live in a space, derive a sense of belonging from the place and make it their base by taking responsibility for it (Kelly and Sewell 1988: 49). Drawing on such a framework enables us to imagine the *base* dimension of community-based education and training as signifying that a group of people have decided to take some responsibility for a space/place. They are not just located at the grassroots –

a colloquial way of talking about local-level community concerns – but are also responsible actors within this grassroots location.

Having provided some settings as to how we understand community as dialogue and a particular kind of collectivity, and also clarifying the 'base' of community as linkages at the grassroots with people taking responsibility, we now turn to the concepts of education and training.

Community-based *Education* and *Training*

As alluded to within the Introduction, it is the combination of both the learning *and* action elements that highlight the meaning of education and training within this book. Also, when referring to action the focus is not on technical or vocationally-oriented action but more radically-oriented action. The integration of learning and action within a radical tradition of education and training has been articulated in an accessible way to community workers by Hope and Timmel (1984), and recently reclaimed by Brookfield and Holst (2011). The latter go on to argue that the 'term training has suffered a downgrading to the point that…many adult educators in North America [and elsewhere]…avoid using the word' (Brookfield and Holst 2011: 66). In tackling this avoidance head on, and as part of reclaiming the radical idea of training, Brookfield and Holst (2011) take the time to both review the many contemporary narrow definitions of what is generally considered to be training today, and then to also overview historical and contemporary examples of training within the radical tradition.

Brookfield and Holst (2011) note that training is often used within discourses of vocational and workplace training. The focus of such training is often on instruction and the underpinning philosophy is usually a neoliberal political economy, that is, training needs are driven by employer needs. In contrast, an alternative reading of the training landscape provides examples of training being used within the radical tradition – often focused more on democratic and participatory processes. For example, Brookfield and Holst (2011) discuss, among others: the Highlander Folk School with its focus on leadership training and training for citizenship; the Citizenship Schools of the 1960s and their training of teachers; the Sandinista National Literacy Crusade in Nicaragua, focused on training local people and local leaders; and Brazil's Landless Workers Movement, with its training of people in co-operatives.

In distilling the practices of such a radical training tradition they identified the following key themes:

- training as the mastery of action (practice) and the mastery of principle (theory) conceived dialectically
- a central element is affective and relational – building the skills, understanding, and confidence of people

- a significant amount of training takes place in the actual activities of social movements: it is training in action
- training is a mutual relationship where both the trainer and the trainee are trained
- training is participatory and democratic in methodology
- training is not neutral: it is oriented to serving the needs of specific sectors of society; it attempts to advance social change activism towards a more participatory and democratic society; it is, therefore, as much a political act as it is a pedagogical act (Brookfield and Holst 2011: 85).

This description of key practices resonates well with our perspective of training and education practices.

It should also be said that many community development processes implicitly hold both processes of community learning and action. Indeed, the stories of Parts II and III of this book might for many feel like, or read like, community development or community mobilisation stories (which they are). However, this book emphasises work that makes the learning *explicit* within the action processes, hence another reason for our reclamation of the notion of training. There is a mandate to train; to make learning integral to the process of acting. Community practitioners using a reclaimed understanding of a radical tradition of education and training processes are concerned with how a collective of people (noting our previous caveat about collectives) are learning, and then translating that learning into action. Community-based education and training is infused and enthused with an ethos that is both learning *and* action-oriented.

At this point the kind of community learning and action that community-based education and training might lead to has not been discussed. In many ways, this will be determined by the mandate of the trainer and the kind of framework that a trainer is drawing on. The different stories of Parts II and III will contextualise different approaches available to the practitioner and provide a sense of the diverse kinds of learning and action that can emerge. However, for the purposes of this chapter we will explain or deconstruct one simple framework that captures the types of knowledge and the roles of educators or trainers that guide much community-based learning.

Types of Knowledge

Patricia Cranton's delightful book *Understanding and Promoting Transformative Learning* (2006) introduces readers to Habermas's (1971) work on knowledge and its application to transformational learning. Her re-articulation of Habermas's work provides us with a useful framework for thinking about the kinds of knowledge being generated that would be driving the collective learning and action process within community-based work. The Habermas framework considers three types of knowledge: technical; practical and emancipatory. Each is discussed in turn and is considered in the light of what we have said previously.

Technical knowledge, sometimes named instrumental knowledge, is focused upon learning a concrete and technical skill. Often there are some kinds of scientific laws embedded within this kind of knowledge. If, for example, a group of people who have come together for collective action around a common concern decide that their action requires learning computer skills, then this could be conceptualised as the acquisition of a technical set of skills. Or, to take another example, if a group of people as part of their action, were designing a longer-term project and decided they needed some training in budgeting skills, then the focus would again be on technical knowledge acquisition. Often people in community development processes ask for technical training, for example, around farming, horticulture, animal husbandry and health or to do with the maintenance of equipment. We can think of this kind of knowledge as important, in the sense that without those technical skills the collective actions might collapse. In and of itself this kind of technical knowledge certainly can contribute to personal growth, in that acquiring computer skills and budgeting skills are highly useful for individuals in negotiating the social world. However, unless applied purposefully within a collective action process such skills do not contribute to collective change processes.

Again, it should be noted that we have previously critiqued a tradition of instrumental education and training that focuses on technical knowledge. What should now be clear is the problem is not with technical knowledge – we all need this in many ways. The problem occurs when technical knowledge is transferred within an instrumental approach focused on vocational or workplace agendas and underpinned by a neoliberal political economy. In a sense then, we are not only reclaiming education and training for more radical purposes, but also technical knowledge for transformative agendas!

Habermas's second knowledge type, practical knowledge, sometimes known as interpretive or communicative knowledge, is the kind of knowledge based on our need to understand each other through language. There are no scientific laws governing communication between people, rather there is always an interpretive process at work. Examples of such knowledge, often found within community-based education or training processes, are: communication skills, conflict-resolution skills, cooperative skills and so forth. There are no natural or scientific ways of communicating, conflicting or cooperating. Such human-relations skills are shaped culturally and contextually. However again, such knowledge and skills are often significant in collective action. Returning to the stories of our Introduction: the Filipino people needed nonviolent conflict negotiating-resolution skills to stand up against Marcos and the military; or within the work of Father Arizmendi in Mondragón people needed to learn about cooperation as a pre-cursor for initiating co-operatives.

Finally, Habermas's third knowledge type, emancipatory knowledge, is knowledge gained through a process of critically questioning ourselves and the social systems we live in. Its philosophical foundations are within critical theory.

Clearly, such knowledge generation is a part of many community-based learning processes. Reflecting on two stories from our Introduction mentioned above; people would not have been able to consider the need to resist Marcos within the Philippines, or imagine the alternative economic practices of co-operatives, unless there had been some kind of emancipatory knowledge acquisition. Within the first story emancipatory knowledge enabled Filipinos to think about the importance of practicing democracy and human rights; and in the second story emancipatory knowledge enabled future co-operators to reflect on the ecological, economic and social consequences of capitalism and to imagine an alternative.

Such a framework of knowledge enables community development practitioners to give careful and conscious consideration to what they are trying to achieve in learning processes. The different kinds of knowledge – technical, practical and emancipatory – are all essential to a radical education/training praxis that enables social learning, organising and mobilisation to take place within community development work.

Role of Educator/Trainer

The knowledge framework described above also helps to distil the different kinds of roles that are adopted by a community-based educator/trainer. Table 1.1 depicts the different roles aligned with the knowledge type.

Table 1.1   Knowledge types and roles

Knowledge type	Role of educator/trainer
Technical	*Instructor:* selects content, orders the content into an agenda, selects materials, and presents.
Practical	*Facilitator:* acts as a resource person, or mentor and model. Trainer builds trust with learners, helps challenge assumptions.
Emancipatory	*Reformist, co-learner, provocateur:* enables groups to see and gain power, which may result in personal and social change.

Clearly, when considering community-based learning processes an educator/trainer needs to be clear about the type of knowledge that might be generated and their accompanying role. There might well be shifts in knowledge type and role as a process changes, but the key is being conscious during shifts and when working in one mode.

Aligned to the questions of knowledge type and the educating/training role is the question of which community development tradition a practitioner is operating from. These are connected issues. A tradition should deeply influence the kind of knowledge being sought and generated, and the political stance taken as an educator/trainer. This idea of community development traditions is now discussed.

Locating Our Practice within Different Intellectual Traditions of Community Development

For us, the notion of community development *tradition* is a gift to community development practitioners-theorists because it provides some clarity about the historical roots and ideological assumptions sitting within different community development approaches. Furthermore, being clear about roots and assumptions links practitioners into a past, present and future 'community of practice', that shares a tradition. Such a community of practice ensures that community development practitioners-theorists are not on a subjective journey, discovering their own individually constructed practice, but are linked into a collective project.

In exploring this idea of traditions we turn to Campfens (1997) who provides a useful framework. In reviewing the many disparate intellectual traditions that underpin the field of community development he categorises them into the broader traditions of societal guidance, social mobilisation and social learning, based upon their key agenda for society. This approach groups various intellectual families into an overarching tradition based upon their core normative agendas, assumptions and prescriptions about social change.

Firstly, the *societal guidance* agenda of community development is underpinned by the 'power of technical reason'. Exemplified by Rostow (1960), practitioners-theorists within this tradition tend not to question existing power relations. They are sometimes known as 'institutionalists', focusing on weaknesses of existing organisations and institutions to deliver a 'programme of development'. Within a community development process informed by such a tradition, community-based education and training focuses on the role of learning in furthering the 'agenda' of a development programme, of either the state or non-state actors. For example, if the state decides that developing small businesses is the best way to enhance community economic development they would 'roll-out' a training programme on 'how to develop and run small businesses'.

Secondly, there is the *social mobilisation* agenda of community development. For Campfens (1997) within this overarching family are a further three categories. Within social mobilisation there is 'confrontational politics' reflected in the work, for example, of Saul Alinsky (1946, 1971). There are the 'politics of engagement', reflected in the Utopian work of activists such as Robert Owen, which has inspired intentional communities and co-operatives (de Schweinitz 1943, Owen and Claeys 1991). And finally, there are the 'politics of free association and mutual aid' reflected in the work of social anarchists such as Proudhon (1979) and Kropotkin (1989). Their work contributed to the advent of self-help groups and local-economic development societies, and the growth of the communitarian movement. Within community development underpinned by this family of social mobilisation traditions, community-based education and training focuses on supporting people's confrontational, engaged or mutuality practices.

Thirdly, the *social learning* agenda of community development draws on a diversity of practices and ideas. These include American empiricism, particularly the pragmatism of John Dewey (1946, 1963); 'action learning' and organisational development; Mao Zedong's essay *On Practice* (1968); popular education, particularly as theorised and practiced by Paulo Freire (1970); liberation theology with its preferential 'option for the poor'; and finally; reconstructing the 'development expert' within social learning. Within the social learning agenda, community-based education and training focuses on the role of learning in supporting the development of such critical consciousness.

Drawing on more recent thinking within the social learning tradition, our perspective of practice also refers to the work of people such as Margaret Wheatley, Allan Kaplan and Robert Chambers. We have been particularly drawn to Wheatley's thinking around complex systems theory (2006), Kaplan's consideration of organic and ecological practices (1996, 2002, 2005) and Chambers's paradigm of adaptive pluralism (2010). Such thinking locates community journeys in learning within a broader paradigm that confronts reductionist and instrumental development practices. The stories told within Wheatley and Freize's recent book *Walk Out Walk On: A Learning Journey into Communities Daring to Live the Future Now* (2011) well illustrates an alternative tradition of thinking and social practice. Within such a community development approach, we would understand community-based education and training as processes that enable social emergence and creativity, imagination and inventiveness, as well as mutual and horizontal learning.

As authors and practitioners, we are more aligned towards the latter two traditions; focused on community-based education and training processes that support, or are a part of, the social mobilisation and social learning agenda for social change. This is not to say that we are opposed to the social guidance tradition, certainly we have 'provided training' within programmes of development and understand its usefulness. However, such work is not the focus of this book.

Conclusion

Community development praxis, requiring interplay between theory and practice, often requires a learning space to consider new theories and choose different practices. Community-based education and training is focused on these created learning spaces that lead to effective engagement with new theory and choice of practices. As demonstrated through this chapter, our philosophical understanding of such a learning space is underpinned by particular notions of 'community as dialogue'. It is a learning space principally aimed at enabling people to build mutual relationships through an exchange of stories, ideas, new thinking and possible concrete actions. As such, it is a humanising space characterised by subject-subject oriented relationships, rather than instrumental space characterised by subject-object relationships. Within such a dialogical space different kinds of knowledge will be mobilised by a group of people – we have named them as technical, practical and emancipatory knowledges. Furthermore, often an educator/trainer will take on an invited and mandated role to animate such a space. The base of such community learning is a connection at the grassroots either directly, or mediated through the horizontal or vertical relations of people's organisations. This base is fundamentally about people taking responsibility for their lives, with a view of education and training as a critically enabling process of collective social learning and social mobilisation.

With such a perspective in mind, we now turn to the next chapter which examines the diverse traces of educational theory that underpin community-based learning.

References

Alinsky, S. 1946. *Reveille for Radicals*. Chicago: University of Chicago Press.

Alinsky, S. 1971. *Rules for Radicals: A Practical Primer for Realistic Radicals*. New York: Random House.

Brent, J. 2009. *Searching for Community: Representation, Power and Action on an Urban Estate*. Bristol: The Policy Press.

Brookfield, S.D. and Holst, J.D. 2011. *Radicalizing Learning: Adult Education for a Just World*. San Francisco: John Wiley.

Buber, M. 1947. *Between Man and Man*. London: Routledge & Kegan Paul.

Buber, M. 1958. *I and Thou*. New York: Charles Scribner's Sons.

Buber, M. 2002. *Between Man and Man*. London: Routledge.

Campfens, H. 1997. *Community Development Around the World: Practice, Theory, Research, Training*. Toronto: University of Toronto Press.

Chambers, R. 2007. From PRA to PLA and pluralism: Practice and theory. *IDS Working Paper 286*. Sussex: Institute of Development Studies.

Chambers, R. 2010. Paradigms, poverty and adaptive pluralism. *IDS Working Paper 344*. Sussex: Institute of Development Studies.

Cranton, P. 2006. *Understanding and Promoting Transformative Learning: A Guide for Educators of Adults*. San Francisco: Jossey-Bass.

de Schweinitz, K. 1943. *England's Road to Social Security: From the Statute of Laborers in 1349 to the Beveridge Report of 1942*. Pennsylvania: University of Pennsylvania Press.

Dewey, J. 1946. *The Public and its Problems: An Essay in Political Inquiry*. Chicago: Gateway Books.

Dewey, J. 1963. *Experience and Education*. London: Collier-Macmillan.

Freire, P. 1970. *Pedagogy of the Oppressed*. New York: Herder and Herder.

Habermas, J. 1971. *Knowledge and Human Interest*. Boston: Beacon Press.

Hope, A. and Timmel, S. 1984. *Training for Transformation: A Handbook for Community Workers*. Zimbabwe: Mambo Press.

Kaplan, A. 1996. *The Development Practitioners' Handbook*. Chicago: Pluto Press.

Kaplan, A. 2002. *Development Practitioners and Social Process: Artists of the Invisible*. Chicago: Pluto Press.

Kaplan, A. 2005. Emerging out of Goethe: Conversation as a form of social inquiry, *Janus Head,* 8(1), 311–34.

Kelly, A. and Burkett, I. 2008. *People Centred Development: Building the People Centred Approach – Dialogue for Community Engagement.* Australia: The Centre for Social Response.

Kelly, A. and Sewell, S. 1988. *With Head, Heart and Hand: Dimensions of Community Building.* Brisbane: Boolarong Press.

Kropotkin, P. 1914/1989. *Mutual Aid: A Factor of Evolution.* Montreal: Black Rose Books.

Kumar, S. 2002. *Methods for Community Participation: A Complete Guide for Practitioners.* London: ITDG Publishing.

Owen, R. and Claeys, G. 1991. *A New View of Society and Other Writings.* United Kingdom: Penguin Classics.

Proudhon, P.-J. 1979. *The Principle of Federation.* Toronto: University of Toronto Press.

Rostow, W. 1960. *The Stages of Economic Growth: A Non-Communist Manifesto.* Cambridge: Cambridge University Press.

Westoby, P. and Owen, J. 2010. The sociality and geometry of community development practice. *Community Development Journal,* 45(1), 58–74.

Wheatley, M.J. 2006. *Leadership and the New Science: Discovering Order in a Chaotic World.* San Francisco: Berrett-Koehler Publishers.

Wheatley, M.J. and Freize, D. 2011. *Walk Out, Walk On: A Learning Journey into Communities Daring to Live the Future Now.* San Francisco: Berrett-Koehler Publishers.

Zedong. M. 1968. On practice, in *Four Essays on Philosophy.* Beijing: Foreign Languages Press.

Chapter 2

Tracing a Tradition of Community-based Education and Training

Lynda Shevellar and Peter Westoby

Tracing the Path

Having explored what we mean by 'community-based' and 'training', and locating this work within a broader context of community development practice, we now turn our attention to the rich educational history that informs our understanding of community-based education and training. Within this chapter we 'trace a tradition' of community-based education and training examining key authors, texts and ideas.

We deliberately use the word 'trace' in the sense of a path formed by the passage of people before us. The path is not linear, but curves and branches and circles upon itself. It has been created over time by walking in each other's footsteps. The fields of education, training and development are vast and to some extent, the boundaries we have drawn here must be arbitrary. However, to create order in an untidy universe, we have categorised three key literatures that inform our understanding of community-based education and training. These are the literatures of adult learning, popular education and transformational learning. It is these three paths of theory and practice that we now explore.

Adult Learning

Many readers will be familiar with the word 'pedagogy': a term used to describe the art and science of teaching. What is less well known is its origins in the monastic schools of Europe in the Middle Ages. Monks taught young boys under a system that required children to be obedient, faithful and efficient servants of the church (Knowles 1984). Pedagogy is derived from the Greek word 'pais', meaning child and 'agogos', meaning leading (although interestingly the Greek word 'pais' also means slave!). Thus, pedagogy has been defined as the art and science of teaching children. In the pedagogical model, the teacher has full responsibility for making decisions about what will be learned, how it will be learned, when it will be learned and if the material has been learned. It is a model that promotes dependency upon the teacher, as the underpinning assumption is that learners need only what the teacher decides to teach them (Knowles 1984).

The pedagogical model has been applied equally to the teaching of children and adults, and the term tends to be used to refer to the art and science of teaching in a very general sense. However, as early as 1833, there was a distinction made between the teaching of adults and children. In a discussion of Plato's educational ideas, a high-school teacher by the name of Alexander Kapp employed the word 'andragogy' to describe the lifelong necessity to learn (Henschke 2005). The term did not come into popular usage until the 1950s where it re-emerged in Germany with the work of Franz Poggeler, and was then picked up by adult educators in Germany, Austria, the Netherlands, and Yugoslavia to describe the method by which adults keep themselves intelligent about the modern world (Knowles 1989: 79). In 1968 in North America, Malcolm Knowles published his first article about his understanding of andragogy with the provocative title *Andragogy, not Pedagogy!* Knowles is widely recognised as the pioneer of andragogy as a specific theoretical and practical approach to learning. For Knowles, andragogy is based on a humanistic conception of self-directed and autonomous learners with teachers as the facilitators of learning. Knowles defines self-directed learning as: 'The process in which individuals take the initiative, with or without the help of others, in diagnosing their learning needs, formulating learning goals, identifying human and material resources for learning, choosing and implementing learning strategies, and evaluating learning outcomes' (1980: 7).

The idea that, given the right environment, people can learn and be self-directed in the way learning is applied is not new and has been an important humanistic theme that can be followed through the philosopher Heider, phenomenology, systems thinking, double loop and organisational learning, andragogy, learner managed learning, action learning, capability and work-based learning (cited in Hase and Kenyon 2000). Consistent with these ideas, Knowles (1970, 1980) sees andragogy as premised upon four key assumptions:

- teachers have a responsibility to help adults in the normal movement from dependency toward increasing self-directedness
- adults have an ever-increasing reservoir of experience that is a rich resource for learning
- people are ready to learn something when it will help them to cope with real-life tasks or problems, and
- learners see education as a means to develop increased competence.

Two additional assumptions were later added (Knowles, Holton, and Swanson 1998):

- adults need to know the reason to learn something
- the most potent motivators for adult learning are internal, such as self-esteem.

Table 2.1   Comparing pedagogy to andragogy

	Pedagogy	Andragogy
Learner's role	Follow instructions Passive reception Receive information Little responsibility for learning process	Offer ideas based on experience Interdependent Active participation Responsible for learning process
Motivation for learning	External: Forces of society (family, religion and so forth) Learner does not see immediate benefit	From within oneself Learner sees immediate application
Choice of content	Teacher controlled Learner has little choice or no choice	Centred on life or workplace problems expressed by learner
Method focus	Gain facts and information	Sharing and building on knowledge and experiences

Source: Used with permission from The Center for Development and Population Activities (CEDPA), 1994: 9.

Table 2.1 captures the key differences between the pedagogical and andragogical learning approaches. It illustrates that, as opposed to traditional educational approaches, the key normative characteristics of adult learning, as defined by Knowles include its voluntary nature and the importance of self-direction. Adult learning places emphasis upon experiential learning predicated on the assumption that adults have issues they want to apply their learning to, and that are relevant to their experience. Within adult learning, the learning style is collaborative and participatory, for example, sitting in circles and working in groups (although some new theorising calls these into question – see, for example, Imel and Tisdell 1996 and Imel 1998b). There is an emphasis on the rich experiences and resources adults bring to learning and the importance of 'self-concept' that is seen as central to a sense of learner empowerment. Adult learning also recognises people learn in different ways and therefore, good learning processes are diverse enough to engage with diverse learning styles. Finally adult learning places value on everyday learning for teaching the fundamental skills of human relations. According to Knowles (1950), this fact makes the task of every leader of adult groups real, specific, and clear: every adult group, of whatever nature, must become a laboratory of democracy, a place where people may have the experience of learning to live cooperatively.

Although andragogy is often cited in education texts as the way adults learn, the term has taken on broader meaning since Knowles's first definition. Marcia Conner asserts that the term currently defines an alternative to pedagogy and is now used to refer to a learner-focused education for people of all ages (Conner 1997, 2004).

Andragogy, and the work of Knowles, are not without criticism. One of the most important critiques has been developed by Daniel Pratt (1993), who questioned Knowles's assumption that all adult learners were willing to engage in a highly participatory and democratic teaching/learning transaction grounded in a Western male concept of individuality. However, Patricia Cranton (2006) observes that Knowles originally theorised adults as having a 'preference' for self-directed learning. In Knowles's original thinking, self-directed learning was not meant to be an isolated or independent means of learning, nor was it intended to describe a personal characteristic as has become the norm. However, the cultural component of the criticism is worth noting.

Similarly, criticisms have been raised by feminists for overlooking gendered structures of power in education (Tisdell 1998) and by critical theorists for putting forward an oversimplified view of individual freedom (Grace 1996). There are also concerns about the evidence base and interpretations of the six assumptions (Rachal 2002) as outlined earlier. Adult learning has also been accused of being narrowly focused on educational technique and course provision (Foley 1999: 2). Finally, contemporary learning theories, such as 'communities of practice' (Wenger 1998) directly challenge Knowles's approach by de-emphasising individual learners. Cranton (2006) acknowledges that despite the origins of adult learning being located in the social change of the 1920s and 1930s, in recent decades there has been a move away from social issues toward an emphasis upon individual learning. Alongside this, Hase and Kenyon (2000) suggest that andragogy is still teacher directed learning. They posit the term 'heutagogy' to better capture the concept of truly self-determined learning. Despite Knowles's claim that the framework can be applied to any adult learning setting, these critiques make it essential to recognise that andragogy only addresses certain types of learning at certain times.

In spite of these critiques, it is clear that the broad body of knowledge that has moved from teacher-led to student-centred learning and from purely theoretical to applied, experiential and interactive education is an important discourse relevant to any formation of a theory of community-based education and training. We also argue that the weaknesses of the andragogic approach are offset by the other traditions we trace – and which will now be explored.

Popular Education

The second tracing along the community-based education and training path is 'popular education'. Popular education is a form of adult education that encourages learners to examine their lives critically and take action to change social conditions (Kerka 1998). It is 'popular' in the sense of being 'of the people'. This is in contrast to the elites of a community, such as big business, political parties and ruling classes. Rick Flowers (2004) refers to this as the distinction between 'education *for* the people' and 'education *by* and *with* the people'.

Although it has been wryly observed that popular education seems to be whatever a popular educator does (Poertner 1994), an extensive paper aimed at defining popular education identifies four main expressions of popular education (Flowers 2004). These are: working-class education in the eighteenth and nineteenth centuries; progressive and radical education; adult education for democracy in the early twentieth century and Freire and his 'pedagogy of the oppressed' which we will discuss in greater detail below.

Popular education shares with the adult learning tradition a participatory pedagogy. So for example, within popular education everyone teaches and learns, thus leadership is shared. It begins with the experiences and concerns of the learners. There is both the creation of new knowledge and critical reflection. However, popular education departs from adult learning and more formal education processes because it has a deliberately political agenda. The goal is to develop 'people's capacity for social change through a collective problem-solving approach emphasising participation, reflection, and critical analysis of social problems' (Bates 1996: 225–6). Brookfield (2005) has provided a useful summary of how critical theory informs liberating education. The task of critical theory is to challenge ideology; confront hegemony; unmask power; overcome alienation; learn liberation; reclaim reason and practice democracy. Thus, popular education explicitly works for empowerment; it aims for social change and has political action as an integral part of its intention (Arnold, Barndt, and Burke 1985; Mackenzie 1993; Wagner 1998). The intention is for people alienated from their own cultures to become self-aware political subjects (Freire 1970; Hernandez 1985, cited in Hamilton and Cunningham 1989: 443). It is this use of critical theory which firmly locates popular education at the crossroads of politics and pedagogy.

Flowers (2004) attests that popular education practice in the Freirean or radical and progressive education sense, goes beyond responding to people's needs and helps people assert their rights. He argues that it does more than promote active participation – as adult learning might do. It fosters robust debate, encourages questioning, fosters a sense of indignation and anger and at times supports confrontation. Popular education does more than help people feel more informed, responsible and self-reliant. It helps people to take action and actively pursue alternative visions for the future. It helps people not just feel empowered but actually strive for *more* power.

Perhaps the most well known expression of popular education lies with Paulo Freire and his literacy work in Brazil in the 1960s. Freire did not develop popular education, but he certainly popularised it and its profound influence on the South American political landscape. Beginning with a deep awareness of the connection between knowledge and power, Freire conceptualises literacy education as far more than learning to read words; rather it is learning to read and name the world itself. His methods are reflexive and dialogical and recognise the power of the facilitator. Welded to this is a profound respect for his students. He does not see them as *tabula rosas* (blank slates) or empty vessels to be filled up. His role rather is to help them decode their world through language; helping them to understand their conditions of poverty not as an *a priori* state of affairs, but as something constructed and reinforced by the actions and power of others, and also by their own inaction.

Pedagogy of the Oppressed (1970) announces the main themes of Freire's career: the non-neutrality of education; the power of knowledge; the coercive force behind rote learning and 'banking' education; the need for dialogical pedagogies; empowerment of the learner and the importance of co-constructing knowledge in the classroom based on the experience of learners. These themes lead to a 'consciousness-raising' or 'conscience awakening'; helping people to see their positionality in the world and to recognising how their knowledge gives them the power to act and to change that world. Freire's philosophy is captured eloquently by Richard Shaull in the introduction to Freire's work:

> Education either functions as an instrument which is used to facilitate integration
> of the younger generation into the logic of the present system and bring about
> conformity or it becomes the practice of freedom, the means by which men and
> women deal critically and creatively with reality and discover how to participate
> in the transformation of their world. (Shaull in Freire 2006: 34)

Freire's work had provided the basic pedagogical concepts and methodologies necessary to stimulate 'critical consciousness' and the transformation of worldview. However, *Pedagogy of the Oppressed* is written in both strongly Marxist and patriarchal language which can alienate some readers. Freire himself suggests that no one can fully understand his ideas from that single text given that his thinking has continued to develop over thirty years. In 1998, Freire wrote *Pedagogy of Freedom: Ethics, Democracy and Civic Courage.* Although he returns to many of his perennial themes, here his vision is wider and more holistic in terms of connecting education with the wider world; to ethics, globalisation, and civil society and in social change. His vision is also more hopeful, reiterating that through critical, reflective pedagogies the world can be transformed into a freer and more just place.

Although Freire's published work did not appear in English until the 1970s, this kind of educational approach has an impressive lineage, most notably Myles Horton's work with the Highlander Folk School during the American Civil Rights Movement, and in Canada with Moses Coady during the Antigonish Movement in the 1930s. Horton created the Highlander Folk School (now Highlander Research and Education Center) in the Appalachian Mountains of Tennessee in the 1930s and worked continually for social justice and transformation until the early 1990s. His lifetime of work played key roles in the American Labor Movement of the 1930s, the American Civil Rights Movement of the 1960s and the environmental and land rights struggle in the Appalachian region in the 1980s. Despite vastly different life paths, the two men shared remarkably similar views and practices on educating for change. Their joint work provides a dialogue that alternates between Freire's conceptual understandings of the connections between education and social change, and Horton's straightforward descriptions of how such ideas have been practiced in reality over six decades (Bell, Gaventa and Peters 1993). Horton emphasises the importance of storytelling for allowing people to share knowledge and build from a collective knowledge-base to address their own problems without being dependent on outside assistance. Freire's complex pedagogical theories are unpacked by Horton's folksy anecdotes about putting those theories into action during his many decades of struggle. This balance of theory and practice illuminates the ideas of transformative learning and demonstrates how it succeeded in changing individuals, and eventually the system itself. While these pedagogies had little impact on mainstream education at the time, they were emphatically accepted in the world of adult education, which also has strong political and emancipatory overtones.

Alongside Freire and Horton, the third author activist who has had a profound influence on popular education is the African American feminist theorist bel hooks. hooks, a former student of Freire, has become a pre-eminent pedagogue in her own right. While embracing Freire's work, hooks (1994: 49) also offers a critique of the sexism of Freire's language and of his patriarchal model of liberation which she read as equating liberation with manhood. hooks adds black feminist perspectives to critiques of education, and also to the way teaching and learning should be re-visioned. hooks, like Paulo Freire, sees education as the practice of freedom and argues that an educator has the 'right as a subject in resistance to define reality' (1994: 53). Her key focus – is on formal academic learning contexts in which she sees teaching as a 'performative act': 'our work is meant to serve as a catalyst that calls everyone to become more and more engaged, to become more active participants in learning'(hooks 1994: 77).

hooks invites us to 'teach to transgress' (1994). By 'transgress,' hooks means to take the standard canon of academic knowledge and interrogate it so deeply, critically and personally that it becomes a radical practice of intellectual freedom. The aim is to expose hidden imbalances of power and unexamined assumptions of embedded ideologies that lie unnoticed in many texts and everyday discourses.

hooks approaches formal education situations and standard classroom topics with such intensity and engagement that the ordinary becomes transformative. For her, the classroom must be a place of energy and excitement: where the educator is responsible for creating the engaged learning environment needed for democratic education. In this context, building energy begins with the teacher and is enhanced by the students; however, it also comes from the teaching material and how it interacts with her students. Because that interaction cannot be anticipated or controlled, hooks says classes that are rigidly planned drain the vitality from the teaching-learning space allowing nothing unexpected to occur. For hooks, facilitating openness where 'conversation is the central location of pedagogy for the democratic educator' (1994: 44) is essential. Teaching to 'transgress' is to step over the line of what a teacher expects, and is expected, to teach; it goes further and deeper with the material and enters the political and personal dimensions of what is being taught. It is a chance to co-operatively deconstruct knowledge and co-create it again. This ability to move beyond the conventional boundaries of teaching, and of the knowledge presented, is the practice of freedom that inspires hooks' work. It is also her technique for consciousness raising, for challenging and provoking her students to undertake a path of personal and social transformation. Such a dynamic and liberated pedagogy requires building a democratic community for learning, one where relationships are fostered so that learners can give voice to both the personal and the controversial.

Although popular education practice can take a wide variety of forms, there is a consistent emphasis placed upon praxis: the interaction of reflection and action. Emerging from people's own experiences a group identifies a common problem. Together people reflect on and analyse the problem, and move between the local and the global, developing theory as they do so. The process is supported by adult educators, or animators, who serve as democratic facilitators, existing in horizontal relationship with the participants. In this context, the educator's role is to keep the group on track; encourage robust participation; ensure that learning takes place and to encourage the development of leadership and self-direction in the group (Arnold and Burke 1983). Educators also assist the group develop a deeper understanding of the problems addressed by placing the issues in a social, historical, and political context (Bates 1996).

Another characteristic of popular education that distinguishes it from other educational traditions is through incorporating popular culture by using drama, song, dance, poetry, puppetry, mime, art, storytelling, and other creative mediums so that 'working class adults recognise their life and their values' (Proulx 1993: 39). In this context, it is assumed that learning is most effective where participation is active, different learning styles are addressed, content is relevant to learners' lives, learners are treated as equals and the learning process is enjoyable (Arnold and Burke 1983). The basic premise is that people who are marginalised have the ability to analyse their own realities and they can be empowered to do so through approaches that emphasise diversity, creativity and the intentional disruption of power relations (Kumar 2002).

It is important to separate popular culture from cultural institutions – often perceived as elitist – as well as from instruments of *mass* culture, such as the media. In popular education learners are active participants, not passive spectators of culture. One of the most dramatic examples of this is participatory theatre, known as 'Theatre of the Oppressed' founded by Brazilian theatre director, writer and politician Augusto Boal (1979). This form of interactive theatre, located in the pedagogical and political principles of Freire, enables audience members to interrupt stories and enact alternatives to explore other ways of understanding and taking action in their world. By using theatre, participants can also act out a situation from real life experience using words, movement, gestures, and props. Similarly, the use of social sculpture and sociodrama allows people to physically position themselves in ways that depict their understanding of an issue or theme. In popular education the intention is to enhance communication among audiences with an oral tradition, demonstrate respect for community cultural values and enhance group spirit, demystify the information conveyed and make it accessible and relevant, and encourage participation and learning by appealing to different modalities (Proulx 1993, Bates 1996).

In thinking about the two literatures traced so far – adult learning and popular education – community-based education and training clearly emerges as a practice steeped in participation, collectivity and an agenda for social change. However, there remains a question about how exactly these techniques empower people to approach their lives differently. To bridge this understanding, we turn to the third path informing our understanding of community-based education and training: that of transformative learning.

Transformative Learning

To pursue the question of how adult and popular education practices assisted people's empowerment, Jack Mezirow and his team of researchers investigated the experience of adult learners who had significant changes in behaviour and mindset because of their learning programmes. As detailed in *Fostering Critical Reflection in Adulthood* (1990), the researchers conclude that critical reflection, where students question the validity of their world-view, is the primary pathway to transformation for adult learners. This process allows students to stand back from their own life experiences, and to deconstruct the meanings they have uncritically given to past events and experiences. Rather than being predicated on a knowledge transfer model, this approach challenges learners existing mental models and schemas. By creating 'disequilibrium' students are encouraged to modify their existing schemas, or at least develop a more nuanced understanding of them (Hedeen, Raines and Barton 2010: 169).

Consciousness-raising, or awakening, through problem-posing pedagogies encourages people to critically reflect upon the things they think they know by looking beneath the surface of their social world. Forces such as the media, constructed social norms, racism and sexism can therefore be understood as socio-cultural 'distortions' which lead people to feel devalued and disempowered. These reflective processes allow learners to reinterpret events more authentically from their own perspective, rather than from socially constructed external forces. By helping to peel away these layers of distortion, learners can begin to see their true positionality in the world and their potential for taking action to address newly perceived power imbalances.

Mezirow holds that a defining condition of being human is the need to understand the meaning of our experiences (Imel 1998a). Here, Mezirow draws on Bourdieu's idea of 'habitus,' in which a person's identity and way of being in the world is shaped by childhood environments and experiences, such that this past habituates inside the person no matter their subsequent circumstances (Bourdieu 1980). Thus, the past structures the present (Bourdieu 1980). For those growing up disempowered by poverty and/or violence and societal conflict, these circumstances can create negative, disempowered self-perceptions about oneself and one's abilities and potentials. Building on earlier transformational education practice, Mezirow formulates techniques and processes for helping learners to unpack and decode these internalised frames of reference. By changing their 'frame of reference,' learners are able to have vastly difference perceptions of themselves and make new more accurate meanings of their lives: meanings that are more empowered, optimistic and engaged. Transformative learning can be therefore understood as the process by which learners 'construe, validate and reformulate the meaning of their experience' (Cranton 1994: 22). They learn how most of their self-perceptions are generated externally to themselves – reinforced by social structures, frequently including educational environments. For Mezirow, this transformative process requires ten clear steps:

- experiencing a disorienting dilemma
- undergoing self-examination
- conducting a critical self-examination of internalised assumptions and feelings of alienation from traditional social expectations
- relating discontent to the similar experiences of others – recognising that the problem is shared
- exploring options for new ways of acting
- building competence and self-confidence in new roles
- planning a course of action
- acquiring the knowledge and skills for implementing a new course of action
- trying new roles and assessing them
- reintegrating into society with the new perspective.

Thus Mezirow defines transformative learning as 'learning that transforms problematic frames of reference – sets of fixed assumptions and expectations (habits of mind, meaning perspectives, mindsets) – to make them more inclusive, discriminating, open, reflective, and emotionally able to change.' (Mezirow 2003: 58).

More recently, the work of Kathleen King has sought to balance Mezirow's highly rational and cognitive approach to transformative learning by focusing on the emotional and ethical dimensions of the transformative experience. She says, 'as [adult learners] wrestle with issues of purpose and meaning, they challenge the core elements of themselves … critical questioning can bring with it self-doubt, fear, anger or happiness' (King 2005: 109). It can be a 'distressing' experience and require difficult choices. The response for learners is not only emotional, but can have physical impacts, as well as consequences for social, family and professional relationships. As King says, 'when learners step into action they are poised on a precipice of risk' (2005: 109). Thus, King's work focuses not only on the experience of the learner but also on the role of the facilitator in providing support for the transformational experience.

Mezirow's work has added sophistication and academic rigour to Freire's earlier ideas about conscience awakening and helped to validate the evolving academic field of transformative education. Today, the processes of transformative learning continue to influence and provide scaffolding for building transformative pedagogies and methods.

Conclusion

The three paths we have traced in this chapter – adult learning, popular education and transformative learning – are not parallel paths, but meander and converge at various points. As a body of work they intersect in their approach to learning and a philosophy of education that underpins our understanding of community-based education and training.

Through adult learning approaches, we explore the role of power in the learning experience, and challenge conventional means of learning and expression. Through popular education, we acquire the idea of 'conscientisation' and of learning as being valued-laden, collectively-developed and political. We understand not only power but empowerment. And through transformative learning, we understand the dynamics that make this possible. However, transformative education theory while powerful in explaining learning processes, suggests a largely personal and private experience. It is only in combination with adult learning and popular education traditions that this process moves from private experience to public expression and from collective learning to collective action. Thus, the paths of adult learning, popular education and transformative learning draw together awareness, empowerment and social transformation that lead to the heart of community-based education and training.

The practice of community-based education and training: how it is applied, practiced and understood, how and where it works, and what its limitations might be is the subject of the remainder of this book.

References

Arnold, R., Barndt, D. and Burke, B. 1985. *A New Weave: Popular Education in Central America and Canada.* Ontario: CUSO Development Education and Ontario Institute for Studies in Education.

Arnold, R. and Burke, B. 1983. *A Popular Education Handbook.* Ontario: CUSO Development Education and Ontario Institute for Studies in Education.

Bates, R.A. 1996. Popular theatre: A useful process for adult educators. *Adult Education Quarterly*, 46(4), 224–36.

Bell, B., Gaventa, J. and Peters, J., eds. 1990. *We Make the Road by Walking: Conversations on Education and Social Change, Myles Horton and Paulo Freire.* Philadelphia: Temple University Press.

Boal, A. 1979. *Theatre of the Oppressed.* London: Pluto Press.

Bourdieu, P. 1980. *The Logic of Practice.* Stanford: Stanford University Press.

Brookfield, S. 2005. *The Power of Critical Theory: Liberating Adult Learning and Teaching.* San Francisco: Jossey-Bass.

CEDPA. 1994. Training trainers for development: Conducting a workshop on participatory training techniques. *The CEDPA Training Manual Series, Volume 1.* Washington: CEDPA.

Conner, M.L. 1997 – 2004. *Andragogy and Pedagogy* [Online: Ageless Learner]. Available at: http://agelesslearner.com/intros/andragogy.html [accessed 9 October 2010].

Cranton, P. 1994. *Understanding and Promoting Transformative Learning: A Guide for Educators of Adults.* San Francisco: Jossey-Bass.

Cranton, P. 2006. *Understanding and Promoting Transformative Learning: A Guide for Educators of Adults.* Second Edition. San Francisco: Jossey-Bass.

Flowers, R. 2004. *Defining Popular Education* [Online]. Available at: http://www.uni-due.de/imperia/md/content/eb-wb/defining_popular_education.pdf [accessed 9 October 2010].

Foley, G. 1999 *Learning in Social Action: A Contribution to Understanding Informal Education.* London: Zed Books.

Freire, P. 1970. *Pedagogy of the Oppressed. New York: Herder and Herder.*

Freire, P. 1998. *Pedagogy of Freedom: Ethics, Democracy, and Civic Courage.* Critical Perspectives Series. Lanham: Rowman and Littlefield Publishers.

Freire, P. 2006. *Pedagogy of the Oppressed, 30th Anniversary Edition.* New York: Continuum.

Grace, A. 1996. Striking a critical pose: Andragogy – missing links, missing values. *International Journal of Lifelong Education*, 15(5), 382–92.

Hamilton, E. and Cunningham, P.M. 1989. Community-based adult education, in *Handbook of Adult and Continuing Education*, edited by S. B. Merriam and P. M. Cunningham. San Francisco: Jossey-Bass, 439–50.

Hase, S. and Kenyon, C. 2000. *From Andragogy to Heutagogy* [Online: UltiBASE] Available at: http://ultibase.rmit.edu.au/Articles/dec00/ hase2.htm [accessed: 9 October 2010].

Hedeen, T., Raines, S.S. and Barton, A.B. 2010. Foundations of mediation training: A literature review of adult education and training design. *Conflict Resolution Quarterly*, 28(2), 157–82.

Henschke, J.A. 2005. Considerations regarding the future of andragogy. *Continuing Education*, 22(1–2), 34–8.

hooks, b. 1994. *Teaching to Transgress: Education as the Practice of Freedom.* New York: Routledge.

Imel, S. 1998a. Transformative learning in adulthood. *ERIC Digest, No. 200.* Ohio: ERIC Clearinghouse on Adult, Career, and Vocational Education.

Imel, S. 1998b. Using groups in adult learning: theory and practice. *Journal of Continuing Education in the Health Professions*, 19(1), 54–61.

Imel, S. and Tisdell, E.J. 1996. The relationship between theories about groups and adult learning groups. *New Directions for Adult and Continuing Education*, 71, 15–24.

Kerka, S. 1998. Popular education: Adult education for social change. *ERIC Digest, No. 185.* ERIC Clearinghouse on Adult, Career, and Vocational Education Ohio.

King, K. 2005. *Bringing Transformative Learning to Life.* Florida: Kreiger Publishing Company.

Knowles, M.S. 1950. *Informal Adult Education.* Chicago: Association Press.

Knowles, M.S. 1968. Andragogy, not pedagogy! *Adult Leadership,* 16(10), 350–52, 386.

Knowles, M.S. 1970. *The Modern Practice of Adult Education: Andragogy Versus Pedagogy.* Englewood Cliffs: Prentice Hall.

Knowles, M.S. 1980. *The Modern Practice of Adult Education: From Pedagogy to Andragogy.* Chicago: Association Press.

Knowles, M.S. 1989. *The Making of an Adult Educator: An Autobiographical Journey.* San Francisco: Jossey-Bass.

Knowles, M.S. and Associates. 1984. *Andragogy in Action: Applying Modern Principles of Adult Learning.* San Francisco: Jossey-Bass.

Knowles, M.S., Holton III, E.F. and Swanson, R.A. 1998. *The Adult Learner: The Definitive Classic in Adult Education and Human Resource Development.* Texas: Gulf Publishing Company.

Kumar, S. 2002. *Methods for Community Participation: A Complete Guide for Practitioners.* London: ITDG Publishing.

Mackenzie, L. 1993. *On Our Feet: Taking Steps to Challenge Women's Oppression: A Handbook on Gender and Popular Education Workshops.* South Africa: Centre for Continuing Education, University of the Western Cape.

Mezirow, J. 2003. Transformative learning as discourse. *Journal of Transformative Education,* 1(1), 58–63.

Mezirow, J. and Associates, 1990. *Fostering Critical Reflection in Adulthood: A Guide to Transformative and Emancipatory Learning.* San Francisco: Jossey-Bass.

Poertner, J. 1994. Popular education in Latin America: A technology for the North? *International Social Work,* 37(3), 265–275.

Pratt, D. 1993. Andragogy after twenty-five years, in *An Update on Adult Learning Theory: New Directions for Adult and Continuing Education, No. 57,* edited by S. B. Merriam. San Francisco: Jossey-Bass, 15–24.

Proulx, J. 1993. Adult education and democracy. *Convergence,* 26(1), 34–42.

Rachal, J.R. 2002. Andragogy's detectives: A critique of the present and a proposal for the future. *Adult Education Quarterly,* 52(3), 210–27.

Tisdell, E.J. 1998. Poststructural feminist pedagogies: The possibilities and limitations of feminist emancipatory adult learning theory and practice. *Adult Education Quarterly,* 48(3), 139–56.

Wagner, P.A. 1998. Popular education in the Philippines: To make ready to risk. *Popular Education Notebook,* 4(1), 20–22.

Wenger, E. 1998. *Communities of Practice: Learning, Meaning, and Identity.* New York: Cambridge University Press.

Part II
Australian Stories of Practice

Chapter 3

'We got to look at our old people, use a different school': Bringing Out Stories Across Generations in the Kimberley

David Palmer

Preface: Ned's Story

This is a story about many old people of the Kimberley. Ned is one of them.

Ned is a *Walmatjarri* bloke who was 'grown up' by senior people in the northern parts of Australia's Great Sandy Desert. He now spends much time in Fitzroy Crossing. This desert country is infamously inhospitable to all but the most seasoned bush people. It is often raging in heat and humidity, extremely remote and uncompromising. In addition, Ned has lost a leg, adding to the challenge of being out bush.

But, Ned loves returning to country. He is often the first in the car on Yiriman Project cultural renewal trips. He loves teaching Indigenous young people in the heat of the day, or having a two-hour conversation at night when everyone else is exhausted. Ned is often the first to get up, singing out for country and rallying people.

This is pretty amazing if you keep in mind that he is a fella who spends most of his time sitting quietly in a place where the whirlwind of town life is whistling back and forth with grog, fighting, lots of emotional pain and 'humbug'.[1]

When Ned is out 'on country' he becomes a boss, asserting his knowledge, his position and his language. He demands respect and ensures that other old people are respected.

However, respect is not a one-way street for Ned. You can see him giving respect when he speaks to young people, often in language, and always in a tone that is soft and kind. He usually does this in *Walmatjarri*, showing that when language gets used you simultaneously hold culture and law, take care of country and look after the old people.

And, like many of his contemporaries he loves to sing on country. He sings to show respect to the old people who came before, passed away and now dwell in country. People wake up to his song. Every night he sings by the fire. When he visits important places he sings. He sings to look after and teach young people. For him it is like going to the movies but better.

---

1   The term 'humbug' refers to antisocial behaviour.

His message to young people is clear. He looks them in the eyes with silence for a few seconds, and then softly says in *Kriol*, 'we are here because we care about you, we have love for you. We know you; you come from a good family. You have a name and you are not no-one walking on the street. You have a big life and a big role to play'.

Ned is one of a number of important educators in the Kimberley, wielding something more powerful than a Certificate IV in Train the Trainer or a university degree in teaching. Ned has country, he has stories and he has family.

Introduction

The Yiriman story comes from the Kimberley region in northwest Australia. The Kimberley itself covers a substantial area approximately twice the size of the Australian state of Victoria. It has a relatively small population with just over 30,000 residents living in the region's six towns (Broome, Derby, Fitzroy Crossing, Halls Creek, Wyndham and Kununnurra) and more than one hundred small Indigenous communities.

People living in the Kimberley experience a climate of extremes – desert temperatures range from close to 0°C at night, to 45°C with high humidity in summer. More than forty per cent who call the Kimberley home are of Indigenous Australian descent. Across the region, at least fifteen language groups with thirty dialects are still spoken.

Much of *Yiriman* country has been relatively isolated from Western influence (apart from the odd missionary, pastoralist or travelling police officer) until the past fifty years. As a consequence, a considerable number of *Karajarri*, *Nyikina*, *Mangala* and *Walmajarri* people have remained close to the country of their ancestors, maintaining culture, language and law more than many other Indigenous Australian groups.

This chapter is about *Yiriman* country, *Yiriman* people and *Yiriman* stories. It provides an account of attempts by Aboriginal communities to support their young people. It offers a story of Elders who are reigniting old systems of education. The chapter describes how desert people think about and carry out, what we often call community-based 'education and training'. In particular, it explores the important part that relationships (skin), place (country) and narrative (story) play in knowledge transfer across generations. In this way, the chapter provides an example of how traditional law and cultural practices have been used to influence contemporary challenges.

The Yiriman Project

Since 2000, the Yiriman Project has worked with young people, their Elders and other generations across the southern Kimberley. It represents attempts by a community dealing with one of the nations' most pressing social challenges: the future for Indigenous young people living in remote Australia.

Yiriman is governed by senior *Karajarri, Nyigina, Mangala* and *Walmatjarri* cultural advisers and is managed by the Kimberley Aboriginal Law and Cultural Centre (KALACC), a non-profit Aboriginal organisation concerned with social and cultural wellbeing. Yiriman started because senior people were 'worrying for' young people who were harming themselves with drugs and 'grog'[2] and getting in trouble with the law. Following long established traditions, they set about organising 'back to country' trips.

The most poetic and illuminating way to understand Yiriman is to listen to how its 'bosses' talk:

> The old people came up with this program called Yiriman to protect and look after kids. When they looking after kids they looking after old people and country same time (John Hopiga).

> We got lots of kids not following our culture, not following mainstream culture, they following lazy culture. Yiriman been stop this lazy culture for ten years now (Anthony Watson).

> What we been talking about is a role model, give young people that confidence, we gonna lift them up to be leaders, so they are next lot to pass things on (Annie Milgen).

> Most of our young people have grown up in town … young people find themselves when they're out bush (Annette Kogola).

> All you gotta do is chuck away that idea that you got somebody over you, you can overcome that. That's why we bringing young people out here to clear their brains to think where they gonna go (John Watson).

> To me Yiriman is a vehicle used in healing our old people and our young people. Our old people know exactly where their grandfather country is. Going there gives them a chance to open up and be kings and queens of their country (William Watson).

The experience of storytelling is the raison d'être for Yiriman elders. It gives them the chance to have their accounts listened to, young people the chance to learn and Aboriginal culture the chance to rejuvenate. In this way, young people become an active part of the stories their parents, grandparents and great-grandparents have featured in while allowing young people's own stories to emerge. Peter Ljubic, the Project's first Coordinator, describes it in this way:

---

2 Alcohol.

> Yiriman is simple. It gives young people opportunities to reconnect and redevelop
> relationships with their old people and with country and build something positive.
> The objective is building stories in young people by providing resources to old
> people to travel out to country and transfer knowledge.

Ex-Women's Coordinator, Michelle Coles, says, 'On country, young people
are listening to the old people, discussing their concerns ... learning more from
elders with each trip to the area' (Taylor 2010: 87–88).

Yiriman also gives people new experiences. They get to visit different
places, work with land management experts, share time with researchers and
scientists, health practitioners, filmmakers and artists. They use new technology,
including digital cameras, video, sound devices and Global Positioning System
(GPS) equipment. This helps build opportunities for self-development, cultural
knowledge transmission, land management work, respect for elders, literacy work
and creative production. As one worker said: 'We use this technology to encourage
the kids to develop profiles of themselves, place and cultural context' (Taylor
2010: 86).

Another feature of Yiriman's work is that trips are carefully planned to
incorporate others such as pastoralists, fire managers, fish scientists, zoologists,
biologists, cartographers, archaeologists, general practitioners, nurses, and
teachers. This has many benefits including providing economic rewards to senior
people, establishing them as knowledgeable and reinforcing their status with
young people (Nesbit, Baker et al. 2001: 191–2).

As Preaud describes, on Yiriman trips young people are reacquainted with
country:

> During a trip, whether on foot or in a car, elders point out salient or meaningful
> features of the landscape which are all fragments of the living body of country.
> This hill which is really a Dog, this tree under which we camped last time, this
> old windmill where your uncle used to work. All this ... gradually builds the
> young people as country themselves. (Preaud 2009: 9)

Western Ideas about Education, Training and Literacy

According to Hull (2003), more conventional approaches to education, start
from the premise that it is essential for members of a community to read and
write in Standard English, succeed against a national set of standards and attain
outcomes that prepare one for the market economy. The task of the educator is to
increase the competency of students. This assumes success equates to a linear and
upward progression. Tied in with this are regular and comparative testing regimes,
administered by qualified and technically authorised researchers/assessors.
Success is measured, with confidence, by standardising research design so that

student achievement is rated against others across the nation. For the purposes of this chapter the term 'Technicist' will be used to describe this style of education.

Those critical of the Technicist approach (Resnick 2002) argue that it focuses too much on retention of ideas taken from outside the community's frame of reference. Additionally, more conventional approaches to education are often overly driven by obsessions about student deficit and the need to contend with educational failure. As Freire (1972) puts it, here education is an exercise much like banking: one starts with an empty, or deficit account, and makes regular small deposits in an attempt to fill what was previously a shortfall in the balance.

An alternative approach to education starts from much broader and more liberal premises. Here competent and functioning community members need a range of skills and knowledge, in addition to reading and writing in English (Warlick 2006: 92). Useful education offers community exposure to a broader range of literacies including: mastering a second language; using new forms of communication technology; experiencing different cultural domains and being able to perform creatively and artfully (Hull 2003). For the purposes of this chapter the term 'Multiple Literacies' will be used to describe this style of education (see also Table 3.1).

Table 3.1   Features of technicist and multiple literacies approaches

Technicist approach	Multiple literacies approach
Literacy = attainment of Standard English	Literacy = discovery for many purposes
Purpose of literacy = preparation for market economy	Purpose of literacy = preparation for life
Focus = reading and writing	Focus = multitude of methods
Assessment of literacy deficits	Encourage multiple literacies of students
Focus = learning outcomes	Focus = process
Measure linear development	Look for quality
Standardised measures assumed culturally neutral	Experiment with new modes of literacy
Test in English	Across languages
Work and test in the classroom	Work and assess in context
Assessed by technician/researcher	Community participation in monitoring

Those working with Indigenous students have long pointed to the limits of conventional education practice (Kral and Schwab 2003, Altman 2009). As Partington (1998: 28) points out, in many Indigenous settings, education is not so institutionalised, contrived and truncated from daily life. Skills are often learned by observation, and by being practiced and acquired through interaction with others, rather than through verbal instruction. Language development and retention is strongly influenced by oral and narrative practice, is memorised across generations and learnt through trial and error (Harris 1980). Social capital is progressed through complex kin relationships that children learn from an early age and develop as they mix with an extended network of family. Formal instruction is usually associated with ritual, on country ceremony, and law and cultural activities. Learning, skill development and literacy are also a lifelong endeavour, with education extending and accumulated throughout the generations (Christie 1992: 45).

As Malcolm (1998) reminds us, those unfamiliar with learning in this context can misinterpret the signs of learning and fail to understand that learners are used to:

- many people speaking at the same time
- attentiveness coinciding with silence or avoidance of eye contact
- adults not talking down to children
- the impoliteness of asking direct questions
- much silence when being addressed (Malcolm 1998: 130).

For those growing up in these settings, reading and writing-based literacy often has less relevance than other forms of literacy, such as spatially focused, aural, visual and artful practice. For example, many Indigenous young people have highly developed musical, spatial and intercultural literacies, and often very quickly developed filmic and photographic literacies (Kral and Schwab 2003).

'Use a different school': Returning to Country

Among Yiriman bosses, the business of teaching their young people is inseparable from country. In part, this is because for *Karajarri, Nyikina, Mangala* and *Walmatjarri* people, country is literally and symbolically an extension of family and self. This reflects long-established ontological traditions that connect the health of country to the health of persons. Deborah Bird Rose (2002: 14) puts it beautifully when she says:

> In Aboriginal English, the word 'country 'is both a common noun and a proper noun. People talk about country in the same way they talk about a person: they speak to country, sing to country, visit country, worry about country, grieve for country and long for country. People say that country knows, hears, smells, takes notice, takes care, and feels sorry or happy. Country is a living entity with a yesterday, a today and tomorrow, with consciousness, action, and a will toward life.

Rose (2004), observes that the process of education on country not only involves the young and their living Elders 'going along together', it also demands a shared relationship with Elders and ancestors long passed away, but still living as spirits as part of country. Important here is the conception that the dead are an integral part of the maintenance of life, as well as the education and experience of the young and living. In other words, the practice of learning on country implicitly involves communion between the young (the living) and the old (the dead). It involves 'paying dues' to the ancestors, respecting the cycle of life in death, and death in life, and learning about their obligations to pass this on to those who 'come behind' (Muecke 1997, 2004).

Working on country is also important because it helps invigorate and make culturally relevant more contemporary practices. For example, since 2006 Yiriman has been supporting women from across the region travel to specific sites to locate plants that grow in various seasons, and pass knowledge across generations. On these trips women demonstrate plant use and tell stories to each other. They also explored bush product and sustainable enterprise possibilities, practicing methods for essential oil extraction, making soap, ointments, balms and the creation of natural dyes.

Consequently, a range of important things happened. The trips provided a means by which women were able to come together in a peaceful way and share wisdom about the environment. They practiced leadership in a safe way, built new skills and combined old knowledge and new technologies. This helped build a very important and special learning environment with senior, middle-aged and young women, sharing the transmission of knowledge. This provided significant moments in which older women could see the fusion of their wisdom with new knowledge from a fast and changing world. All of this occurred in an environment where young adults were leading and mentoring teenage women, with Elders looking on.

Michelle Coles described the importance of country in helping with this 'integrated learning':

> Annie is a senior woman who has a heartfelt desire to see knowledge about plants and medicines transferred from generation to generation. She knows young people need to engage with the broader community, with town life. She said, 'I want to find out how to make products from using our plant medicine'. This is a time consuming process. Annie is a health nurse who works like everybody else ... Culture requires her elders are with her when she is making medicine ... she needs to have younger women and thirty and forty year old women alongside her. This learning and teaching space is very different to a school or TAFE because it is on country and with family.

'Gotta know your skin': 'Holding' Young People

Another feature of Yiriman is that it incorporates learning about traditional kinship obligations into its work on country. This reflects the continued importance of 'skin groups' across the generations; between language groups and in teaching young people respect and responsibility.

In the Kimberley, indeed across many regions of Australia, Indigenous people are divided by birth into different groups. These groups have specific names and cross language groups, state borders and regions. One's 'skin', automatically established by birth, allows people to know how to relate to others over an extended family network. Within this system, some groups are considered 'straight skins', able to marry or be close to each other. In addition, skin orders relationships across generations, determining the conduct of important ceremonies, particularly during what is called 'law time'.

These skins, referred to by anthropologists as sections and subsections, indicate generational and sexual divisions so that a parent and their children belong to different groups, as does a husband and wife. It means that children and young people are 'grown up' by a range of people acting as parents. It also means that all Indigenous peoples have large sets of obligations to many brothers and sisters, uncle, aunties, nephews and nieces. Importantly, this system allows outsiders and those new to a community to be recognised, assigned particular responsibilities, and enjoy support and certain rights (see Myers 1991).

Yiriman bosses take seriously the importance of reinforcing young people's knowledge of skin and social obligation. Indeed, 'education work' about skin is often strong during Yiriman trips. This regularly involves a combination of instruction, proximity with certain people and activities carried out in the groups. At the beginning of on country trips, the Elders set about arranging people into their respective skin groups. This is done in conjunction with middle-aged cultural advisers to make sure young people from different towns are included. During the trip, various activities help reinforce and extend people's knowledge of these social systems.

This also helps create conditions where young people feel safe and supported, in a healthy space, able to share openly and honestly in an experience of extended family. As one Yiriman report describes:

> Most nights there are deep discussions about a wide range of topics including language, culture and music, life in town and stories about the day's walk. After the sun goes down the young people rest on swags by the fire, speaking of their personal situations, things that worry them, their contact with the justice system, their desire to change things and their stories of life (cited in Palmer 2010).

This intense love, connection and sense of obligation between young people and their seniors reflect the importance to skin relationships of education work across the generations. Particularly important here is the obligations that come with age to nurture those who 'come along after' (Myers 1991: 211). As a consequence, a regular feature of Yiriman trips and activities is the involvement of three or four generations. As Taylor (2010: 90) observes:

> The young cultural advisers are mentored and trained to take on leadership roles ... senior cultural advisers direct trips on country and establish appropriate

cultural links for specific trips. Middle aged cultural advisers ... liaise with traditional owners and travel identified routes, visiting only the water sources they are allowed, stopping at places with the right people, hunting only with the right people for certain country.

McCoy (2008: 22) describes this process as supporting what *Kukatja* (neighbouring language group to *Walmatjarri*) call *Kanyirninpa*. *Kanyirninpa* is made manifest in a number of ways. It includes both nurturing the young with older people taking responsibility and offering protection. In this way, *Kanyirninpa* involves teaching and learning so that older people help young people grow up the right way.

McCoy (2008: 28), claims that this business of *Kanyirninpa* ('holding' or 'carrying') young people, is an act of exercising 'respect' towards others, creating conditions to reinforce social bonds and social obligations. It is expected that when they get older young people will adopt the same practice and attitude towards their children. As one person puts it, 'if you hold that person, that person will return that respect to you' (cited in McCoy 2008: 18).

'Bringing out stories in young people': Using Narrative

One of the key motivations for establishing Yiriman was to encourage young people to pick up and retell 'stories for country'. At one, and the same time, this experience of storytelling gives Elders the chance to have their accounts listened to, young people the chance to learn and Aboriginal culture the chance to rejuvenate.

'Bringing out the stories' is important in a number of ways. Combining storytelling with tactile and active work both helps senior people recall their lives and give life to young people. Being on country while you talk about country demands people exercise a range of sensory tools. During trips young people listen to the accounts of their Elders while their imagination is enriched by the opportunity to see, touch, smell, and, indeed feel the stories. In this way, storytelling mixed with other forms of learning acts as a form of mnemonics; improving and bringing to a more public forum people's memory of life in the desert.

Storytelling is also an important practical way of challenging young people's tendency to recoil from social interaction with their Elders. By creating spaces for people to tell their stories Yiriman helps people extend the depth of their relationship, build their social repertoire and make new contacts across the region. In other settings, people might describe this act as network building.

Narrative work is also critical because of its ability to call forth, and help people contend with emotions, trauma and difficulties in a safe way. Combining storytelling with camping on country and other activities, like hunting or producing bush products, also allows young people to start to grapple with difficult situations and traumatic events, such as suicides and early death.

In desert life the complex and rich articulation of traditional stories (see Myers 1991, Stanner 2009) connects the past, the present and the future. These accounts emerged from Creation Stories and represent the means through which people learn lessons to assist: conduct, rules for living, relationships, decision-making and sustaining knowledge for future generations.

These stories also allow bosses to nourish the use of *Walmatjarri, Nyikina, Mangala, Karajarri, Kriol* and Aboriginal English. Consequently, the language is often evocative, in part because it is authentic and relevant to the experiences of people, in part because it often involves humour, and in part because it is rooted in figurative speaking.

In this way Yiriman's approach to education and training becomes a means through which young people can become an active part of the stories their parents, grandparents and great-grandparents have featured in. As two senior people remark, this also allows young people's stories to emerge:

> Old people been tell story, young people pick up that story. Future for culture side kids can pick up. Young people love it (Mr Joe Brown).

> Every morning [we] tell 'em the story. What to do in life and out bush. Tell 'em you gotta understand and be real good. Learn some culture (Ned Cox).

One recent trip, a ten-day 150 km walk from the Fitzroy River to the edge of the Great Sandy Desert, was arranged at the instruction of *Nyikina* and *Mangala* bosses. The idea was to take young men on a walk to the place named *Yiriman*; a landmark hill associated with stories about old people from many areas coming together to share law and culture. This place represents a geographical site of importance, a landmark seen from very long distances, a metaphoric lighthouse that acts to guide people towards an area of fertility and sustenance. In this way, the trip was intended as a pilgrimage, a symbolic trip walking young men to meet up with the old people, or spirits, from the past. William Watson described it in this way:

> Yiriman is like a lighthouse for the people from the desert when they came through into our country ... a landmark that showed old people where to pass through to get to this rich country with lots of water, food and stories ... so we backtracked to that place ... we did this to make a story of going back to meet and greet the old people.

As young men walked and camped around fires, they reignited old accounts, making legends with themselves as living actors. In this way, they started practicing to be 'cultural bosses' in the future, extending the legacy of the camp well beyond the life of the trip. As Peter Ljubic remarks, these storytelling opportunities have multiple consequences for the different generations:

The real influence of Yiriman has been in the hundreds of stories that have been created, told and retold. These stories give people a way to share in each other's lives, a way to imagine a future that might be better ... they give people cultural, social and even economic currency. They give guidance to young people trying to find their way, a way for the middle generation to keep things going and the milk and honey that sustains old people and keeps them sparked up.

Others have long recognised the benefits of 'bringing out young people's story'. Storytelling is an important ingredient in the formation of solidarity and community. It is says Kant, what allows humans to enjoy a shareable world (cited in Kearney 2002: 63). Carson suggests a story creates conditions for a cycle of social contact (cited in Kearney 2002: 125). Stories are commonly generated from people doing things together. When told these stories often build relationships between the teller and another group (the audience). The cycle is completed when they are retold. In this way, the story sets up a relationship between a triad that, according to Simmel (1950), is the beginning of community. Every story involves: (i) someone (a storyteller), (ii) telling something (a story about a second person), (iii) to someone else (a listener who becomes the third person) (Kearney 2002: 150).

There is also much evidence that stories can be helpful in healing and therapy, contending with pain and helping sufferers purge and divest their old histories (Parkinson 2009: 45). Storytelling also helps spark imagination and encourages people to think about their world in different ways.

Stories have an important part to play in the transmission of community values, ideas and culture. The Greeks understood this, often using mythology as a way to teach lessons about virtues and ideas about the moral good. In part, this is because stories can communicate abstract principles. In part, it is because a story can establish patterns in human behaviour and evocatively convey a moral idea without appearing to dictate or moralise (Kearney 2002 p. 79). In this way, story is an important ingredient in learning. As Stalling (cited in Kearney 2002: 37) reminds us, an unusually deep form of active stillness can fall upon people during story. This can lead to a true altered state of consciousness that makes one highly susceptible to profound learning and development. As Parkinson (2009: 301) reminds us, 'say worthwhile things in a logical way and they may disappear into the ether. Use an image, tell a story, make an analogy and it wakes people up'.

Conclusion

'Outcomes-based' education has enjoyed over a decade of popularity. Here success has been measured according to market outcomes, against national curriculum standards and by a growing band of policy and research experts. While it has had its advocates and detractors, one thing remains uncontested, during the period when it has shaped national educational and training policy, the gap between Indigenous and non-Indigenous performance has increased (see Holland 2011).

At the same time, there have been a number of experiments with community-driven projects aimed at buttressing quality of life for Indigenous young people. One such experiment has been the Yiriman Project, an innovative attempt at cultural renewal set up by *Karajarri, Nyikina, Mangala* and *Walmatjarri* cultural bosses. The Project draws upon three interconnected elements in traditional desert culture and law: country, skin and story.

In this way, the Yiriman Project provides us with insights into how education and training can use a 'different school', one that combines learning with community, one that draws on ancient and contemporary practice. Lloyd Kwila, one of Yiriman's middle aged 'bosses', points out that this is critical for Indigenous families who are seeking to regain responsibility for family, land and culture:

> Yiriman is like a school for our young people – learning our duty of care for country. When you don't go to country you don't care. It is like a dead heart and weed grows. Young people have a right to know that it is their duty of care to look after country. Yiriman doing a proper good job. Yiriman understand we got to look at our old people, look to country, use a different school.

References

Altman, J.C. 2009. *Beyond Closing the Gap: Valuing Diversity in Indigenous Australia*, Values and Public Policy: Fairness, Diversity and Social Change Conference, Centre for Public Policy, Melbourne University, 26–27 February 2.

Christie, M. 1992. *Aboriginal Perspectives on Experience and Learning: The Role of Language in Aboriginal Education*. Victoria: Deakin University Press.

Freire, P. 1972. *Pedagogy of the Oppressed*. New York: Continuum.

Harris, S. 1980. *Culture and Learning: Tradition and Education in Northeast Arnhem Land*. Darwin: Northern Territory Department of Education.

Hinton, R. 2010. *Shadow Report on the Australian Government's Progress Towards Closing the Gap in Life Expectancy Between Indigenous and Non-Indigenous Australians*. Melbourne: Closing the Gap.

Hull, G.A. 2003. Youth culture and digital media: New literacies for new times. *Research in the Teaching of English, 38*(2), 229–33.

Kearney, R. 2002. *On Stories*. London: Routledge.

Kral, I. and Schwab, J. 2003. The realities of Indigenous adult literacy acquisition and practice: Implications for capacity development in remote communities. *Centre for Aboriginal Economic Policy Research (CAEPR) Discussion Paper D257/2003*. Canberra: CAEPR, Australian National University.

McCoy, B.F. 2008. *Holding Men: Kanyirninpa and the Health of Aboriginal Men*. Canberra: Aboriginal Studies Press.

Malcolm, I. 1998. You gotta talk the proper way: Language and education, in *Perspectives on Aboriginal and Torres Strait Islander Education*, edited by G. Partington. New South Wales: Social Science Press, 57–69.

Muecke, S. 1997. *No Road (Bitumen all the Way)*. Western Australia: Fremantle Arts Centre Press.

Muecke, S. 2004. *Ancient & Modern: Time, Culture and Indigenous Philosophy.* Sydney: University of New South Wales Press.

Myers, F.R. 1991. *Pintupi Country, Pintupi Self: Sentiment, Place and Politics among Western Desert Aborigines.* California: University of California Press.

Nesbit, B., Baker, L., Copley, P., Young, F. and Anangu Pitjantjatjara Land Management. 2001. Cooperative cross-cultural biological surveys in resource management: Experiences in the Anangu Pitjantjatjara lands, in *Working on Country: Contemporary Indigenous Management of Australia's Lands and Coastal Regions,* edited by R. Baker, J. Davies and E. Young. Melbourne: Oxford University Press, pp.187–98.

Palmer, D. 2010. *Opening up to be Kings and Queens of Country: An Evaluation of the Yiriman Project.* Fitzroy Crossing: KALACC. Unpublished report.

Parkinson, R. 2009. *Transforming Tales: How Stories Can Change People.* London: Jessica Kingsley Publishers.

Partington, G. 1998. In those days it was rough: Aboriginal and Torres Strait Islander history and education, in *Perspectives on Aboriginal and Torres Strait Islander Education,* edited by G. Partington. New South Wales: Social Science Press, pp. 27–54.

Preaud, M. 2009. *Earth and Body in Movement: The Contemporary Creation of Aboriginal Countries in the Kimberley.* Unpublished thesis.

Resnick, M. 2002. Rethinking learning in the digital age, in *Global Information Technology Report 2001–2002: Readiness for the Networked World,* edited by G. Kirkman. London: Oxford University Press, pp. 32–7.

Rose, D.B. 2004 *Reports from a Wild Country: Ethics for Decolonisation.* Sydney: University of New South Wales.

Rose, D.B. with D'Amico, S., Daiyi, N., Deveraux, K., Daiyi, M., Ford, L. and Bright, A. 2002. *Country of the Heart: An Indigenous Australian Homeland.* Canberra: Aboriginal Studies Press.

Simmel, G. 1950. *The Sociology of Georg Simmel.* Illinois: Free Press.

Stanner, W.E.H. 2009. *The Dreaming and Other Essays.* Melbourne: Black Inc.

Taylor, F. 2010. *Partnerships in the Youth Sector.* Melbourne: The Foundation for Young Australians.

Warlick, D.F. 2006. Contemporary literacy – the three Es, in *Digital Literacies for Learning,* edited by A. Martin and D. Madigan. London: Facet Publishing, pp. 91–98.

Chapter 4

Poverty Finds a Voice: Dialogic Learning and Research through Theatre in Melbourne

Kathy Landvogt[1]

Introduction

One December day in 2008, in Melbourne's Macquarie Bank headquarters, a group of women performed a series of plays about living on low income. This was the culmination of a theatre project that enabled the women to tell their stories of not having enough money to live with dignity. These stories were the women's critical answer to others' preoccupation with the financial literacy of those living on low income. The event was a purposeful encounter between ombudsmen, bankers and policy makers, and the people that their policies and practices most affected. Responsible for bringing these two worlds together, I straddled the dualities anxiously, knowing what a stark contrast this environment was to the old church hall we had been gathering in. As we escorted the group of ten or so participants through the cathedral-like marble lobby of the bank, a towering Christmas tree greeted us with a sign inviting employees to leave a gift for those less well-off. One participant's exclamation named the surreal moment for all of us: 'Look! Presents for the poor: that's us!' That day, in a performance space more commonly used for corporate presentations, we felt as if we owned the magnificent view over the city. One woman, who had successfully struggled with her agoraphobia to reach the project's many other venues could not face the lift and had to miss the event; and the curtains had to be closed to prevent another having an anxiety attack. These details illustrate the awkwardness of bringing together, through this project, two parallel universes more accustomed to meeting in a charity context.

This story began as research into financial knowledge and poverty, evolved into a participatory theatre project, and eventually wove together training, advocacy, and research in a multi-layered and complex endeavour.[2] Given the critical nature of the research topic, the research method had to be sensitive to the voices that had been silenced in the public discourse of financial literacy, and to empower, rather

---

1   I wish to acknowledge and thank Xris Reardon, Artistic Director of Third-Way Theatre and facilitator of the theatre process in this project, for her input into this chapter, especially the description of the methodology and the ethical framework. For more information about Third-Way Theatre please explore www.thirdwaytheatre.org

2   This project was funded by the Victorian Consumer Credit Fund in 2007.

than marginalise, its participants. Engaging a group of women in a participatory theatre process, we set out to answer the questions, 'What financial education do low income women typically need and how can it best be delivered?' The women produced a rich vein of research evidence, and at the same time were trained as performers and advocates. While participatory theatre is not commonly used as a research methodology, there are previous accounts which demonstrate that research can co-exist with the more direct social change goal of building capacity for self-advocacy (Sloman 2011). The women examined and crystallised their own experiences in 'the money system', learning to see that their experiences were shared, and to critique the economic, corporate and government behaviour that produced those experiences. This approach was in the tradition of other participatory-based theatre, aiming to create 'a bottom-up strengthening of poor people's participation in the policy making and implementation of development' (Sloman 2011: 2).

Community-based education and training, as a tool of social change, is based on structural analysis. The structures this project challenged were the set of beliefs and corresponding public policies which hold poverty to be the result of poor money management and ignorance. These policies and their origins will be briefly outlined before turning to the way in which these were challenged.

The Need for Change

In 2006 large billboards had started appearing across Australia encouraging its citizens to 'understand money' better. Television advertisements delivered messages about budgeting, investing, saving, superannuation and avoiding debt. This was part of the Australian Federal Government's attempt to raise awareness of financial literacy and its benefits, and encourage people to find out more about how to make the most of their money. The media response was, in part, influenced by the flurry of concern in banking and government circles over the results of the first national surveys measuring Australians' financial literacy performance (ANZ and AC Nielsen 2005, Financial Literacy Foundation 2007).

This new policy domain of financial literacy has interesting origins. An uneasy marriage of government and financial services existed in which government allowed the industry a degree of self-regulation provided it did not exploit that freedom.[3] Financial literacy is one child of that pact. The seed had been planted by the Organisation for Economic Co-operation and Development (OECD 2005), but grew in the context of a national government concerned that Australians needed to become more informed financial consumers and better savers for the future. The other catalyst was the financial services industry which, having withdrawn banking services to less profitable customers in the financial services de-regulation of the

---

3   Arguably the national Credit Reform of 2010 (National Consumer Credit Act 2010) shifts that balance of power towards greater protection of the consumer by government.

1990s, was now becoming concerned about financial inclusion. The financial services industry was keen to both expand its markets and improve its image with the public. Financial education was therefore linked to these much bigger, and often regressive, agendas.

National surveys showed that the least well-off members of the community were the lowest on overall financial literacy measures, and banks and government policy makers were targeting low income Australians in their financial education campaigns. The practice experience of Good Shepherd Youth & Family Service, the workplace of the author of this chapter, indicates that people on low incomes are generally excellent money managers who often lack the resources to deal with the financial impacts of disability, mental illness, addiction, separation, domestic violence or simply the rising cost of living. The national surveys also showed low income people to be skilled in day-to-day tracking of expenses, to value saving, and to be debt-averse. While women scored lower overall than men, and showed less future-focus, they clearly face structural barriers to acquiring assets and superannuation; research has identified that women typically put immediate family needs first in financial decisions (WIRE 2007). People living on the bare minimum may well need assistance with negotiating financial matters, but the Australian Government's 'Understanding Money' campaign was not reflecting their lived reality. When financial literacy started to be held up as the panacea to poverty, it was time to weigh into the public discourse with some reality checks about the skills and struggles of those on limited incomes. At the Good Shepherd Youth & Family Service, we decided to undertake research that would add a view from the margins, and encourage governments and community agencies to design financial education programmes based in lived experience.

Along with the structural context, the organisational context is a crucial driver of social change-oriented projects like community-based education and training. In a funding climate that does not generally favour community development activity, this becomes even more important. Good Shepherd Youth & Family Service (2011) has a mission statement that includes the injunction 'to boldly challenge the structures and beliefs that diminish human dignity'. With its roots in nineteenth century France, and now in over seventy countries, Good Shepherd's numerous organisations focus on achieving social justice for the world's poorest, especially women and children. Research and advocacy grounded in practice experience is part of this agenda in Australia. Financial services have been a major focus of the agency's advocacy agenda, especially microfinance programmes, consumer rights and financial regulation.

Using the Living 'Critical Literacy' Tradition of Paulo Freire

In September 2005, Good Shepherd Youth & Family Service organised a discussion with leading microfinance thinker and practitioner Ingrid Burkett[4] about microfinance and financial inclusion. Ingrid noted the burgeoning new orthodoxy of financial literacy, and posed the question, what would financial literacy using Paulo Freire's 'critical literacy' framework look like? Our first response to this challenge was a published paper entitled *Critical Financial Capability: Developing an Alternative Model* (Landvogt 2006). We replaced the term 'literacy' with 'capability' to encompass both the individual's ability and the wider context enabling them to express that ability (Sen 1999). Financial capability is also the term used in the United Kingdom (UK) where extensive research has underpinned its operationalisation (Kempson 2006). The paper presented a 'financial consciousness-raising' model which applied Paulo Freire's critical literacy process (Freire 1972) to financial capability. The model is summarised in Table 4.1.

The theatre training project eventually developed as a practical application of this financial consciousness-raising model. Janet Palafox ibvm,[5] who had worked with Good Shepherd and was familiar with 'Theatre of the Oppressed' (Boal 1979) suggested participatory theatre as a research methodology embodying education and training. Like Ingrid's question a year or so earlier, Janet's suggestion was a well-placed reflection from an experienced community practitioner. Participatory theatre encompasses many variations, but always 'engages people to identify issues of concern, analyse and then together think about how change can happen, and particularly how relationships of power and oppression can be transformed,' (Sloman 2011: 3). Originating in Freire's *Pedagogy of the Oppressed* (1972) and in the work of his followers, especially Augusto Boal (Boal 1992, Paterson 1995), this method allows knowledge and experience to be explored collectively without using written text.

Choosing Freire's *pedagogical* method to double as a *research* method had a pleasing symmetry considering the research question, 'What are the financial information needs of women living on low incomes?' was itself about learning. It certainly satisfied the requirement to take empowerment of the participants seriously. It clearly located the research approach within a broader community-based education and training methodology, ensuring a mutuality of learning between participants and facilitators, and the integration of learning and action. It added complexity but provided an irresistible opportunity.

We engaged Xris Reardon, Artistic Director of Third-Way Theatre (TWT). TWT has its roots in Freire's work and Boal's practice of Theatre of the Oppressed and, therefore, aligned with the theory, method, and ethics of our project. The TWT

---

4   For related information see Ingrid Burkett's publications at Foresters Community Finance at http://www.foresters.org.au/index.php?option=com_content&view=article&id=36&Itemid=25

5   "ibym denotes a Loreto religious sister.

Table 4.1   Application of critical literacy to financial capability

Elements of critical literacy	Application to financial capability
Teaching and learning are part of the same process; teachers are students and students are teachers	Financial counsellors, microcredit workers, and other workers engage as facilitators not as 'experts'
Illiteracy is a concrete example of an unjust social reality, therefore it is political to learn to read	Financial exclusion is due to an unjust social reality, therefore it is political to become financially literate
The way reading is taught should therefore enable students to see the world as 'a limiting situation which they can transform' through identifying social, political, and economic contradictions	Financial education should identify economic contradictions and how they are socially constructed so people can see how change is possible
Learners can see their everyday world afresh through 'codifications', that is, familiar realities showing essential problems or contradictions in everyday lives presented in an unfamiliar form (and therefore not associated with failure)	For example, a codification of 'savings' looking at strategies on a low income such as separate money jars, or a social club kitty, which, proportional to income, may save more this way than other people do in banks
Learners reflect on these codifications by describing them, then 'problematising' them (analysing their deep structure or decoding them) until they see their own lives in that new context	One-on-one or group discussions about Who? What? Why? Appreciating positives in peoples' financial management and problems in society's financial arrangements
Dialogue is the essential type of discussion that this decodification happens within; a synthesis between the educator's and the learner's different types of knowledge	Dialogue between workers and service-users in which workers have 'meta knowledge' (concepts about financial knowledge) and service-users have knowledge of their own lived financial reality
'Generative concepts' (selected words or phrases that have emotional power and leverage to change the way people see the world) are arrived at through dialogue over codification and after careful investigation of the world of the students	Fresh, respectful ways of presenting and dialoguing about financial issues and information will produce the generative concepts; workers alone cannot determine them
Generative concepts are the focus of further dialogue, and are broken down and used to create new concepts	Financial workers continue to use dialogue and learner-based process throughout
This leads to 'conscientisation', the ability to act on the world as subjects	Consciousness of current financial capability skills leads to increase in conscious strategies and self-advocacy with financial services

Source: Landvogt 2006.

philosophy assumes that there are many diverse and complex relationships creating oppression, and that finding solutions to social crises requires understanding the point of view of all the players. It suits the complex social situations of advanced capitalist societies where oppression is harder to trace to one concentrated source than in the developing countries where Theatre of the Oppressed originated.

The method consists of six main stages: identifying the question to be explored by the group; recruiting a group that shares a specific struggle; conducting theatre workshops to devise short plays ending in a moment of crisis; performing the plays to community 'spect-actors', transforming the crisis though spect-actor interventions and creating understanding and change through addressing the struggle. This process is depicted in Figure 4.1.

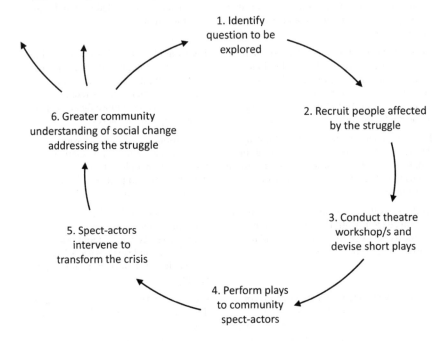

Figure 4.1   The theatre process

The theatre process is one of critical inquiry into the issue and its context. The plays develop from investigations of the individual participants' images created out of exercises, reflection and feedback led by the TWT facilitator. The group's ground rules create respect and listening, with an initial check-in around the group and a closing opportunity to de-brief. The participants recover kernels of experience that have the emotional and symbolic power to drive their story and confront a difficult social issue. This occurs collectively; shared discoveries protect private experience while strengthening the plays' power as social narrative. No one truth can speak for the group, and all present are open to listening deeply to each other. The stories do not reach a resolution, instead they challenge the audience to engage with, and address the problem. In this way, audience members are transformed into participants, becoming 'spect-actors' as Boal names them. Invited by the facilitator, spec-tators are encouraged to stop the play, get up on stage and replace characters whose struggles they understand to try out alternative solutions, or interventions. Through this active participation, or even through witnessing it, spect-actors are moved to join the community of interest created by the play and advocate for change. This process is directed throughout by the facilitator with care for the well-being of participants and audiences, and for the integrity of the story itself.

Creating 'community': Commonality in Diversity

Recruitment of participants is often a challenge in both research and community work. We invited women who had recently received a no-interest loan (NILS®) from Good Shepherd Youth & Family Service and refugees and asylum seekers from Good Shepherd Social Justice Centre. Other women-specific community programmes in the organisation's various locations participated later as audiences. When our quota of up to twenty women fell short we cast the net wider to other disadvantaged community groups previously involved in Third-Way Theatre and women from a local Migrant Resource Centre. We had toyed with the idea of locating the project within a more defined geographic community, but our project had not grown out of any specific agency programme, nor was there an obvious location. Therefore, we drew together a community of women sharing the struggle of living on low incomes. This was consistent with well-accepted views of 'community' as going beyond geography, and certainly was vindicated by the successful outcomes of the project. One disadvantage of the project ending was having no organisational infrastructure to support ongoing community-based education and training with the women, despite the fact that several would have been pleased to continue. This is a comment on the available resources and infrastructure rather than a reflection on the theatre methodology, although it has been noted that a drawback of this method is being time and resource intensive (Sloman 2011).

Xris had spent several months meeting with interested women face-to-face and ensuring they understood the theatre training process and the research question to be investigated. Self-selection into the project was critical to its success and only possible with considerable investment made at the preparatory stage. This process centred on care for the participants and was expressed in a mutually agreed 'ethical framework' document. We were asking for quite a commitment with an initial attendance of six all-day theatre training workshops. To make the workshops as accessible as possible in a central location, we covered transport and child care costs. We provided snacks and lunches, and allowed time for the sharing and informal group interaction essential to community work. All these were part of the philosophy of TWT and the approach of Good Shepherd.

The participants came from all over Melbourne and beyond. The youngest was 20 and the oldest in her sixties. One young woman had been in Australia for six months and used an interpreter throughout. Several participants suffered from mental illness, physical disability or chronic illness. One was a homeless young woman living in a hostel. Several were carers of small children or extended family. Some participants were employed casually and a few were studying, but most were on Australian Government income support payments (Disability Support, Single Parenting Payment, Jobseekers' allowances). The diversity of participants was applauded, but as is common in community development and social learning processes, it was about achieving balance between having enough in common to bond, and enough difference to learn from. Too much difference can make it unsafe to share experiences (Butler and Wintram 1991, Lister 1997). Talking about money broke social norms given that this is a sensitive topic, even a transgressive one in many social situations. For the women participants speaking of personal financial hardship risked exposure to an abject social identity, the shame of failure and being made vulnerable to others' pity and disrespect. It was important to ensure that the women were amongst others who shared similar experiences. Many people complain about not having enough money at some time, but 'not having enough' is relative. A woman working part-time may struggle, but if she has some money in the bank, equity in a home or superannuation, her options are much greater than those of a woman living on a Disability Pension, with none of those assets. The women made the observation that it is difficult to speak honestly about their situation until they can be sure that they are not speaking across too great an experiential gulf.

The group worked hard to develop its collective narratives. The women were very respectful towards each other and this, along with skilful facilitation, built bridges across their difference. The story they felt they all shared was of women pushed to the margins in a money-obsessed society, carrying the burden of social failures, such as poverty, domestic violence and gender inequities.

Speaking Out of Silence

One of the reasons for conducting our research using Third-Way Theatre as a community-based learning experience was to give the participants a clean slate to portray, and so change, their experiences. As Freire said, 'it is in speaking their word that men (sic) transform the world by naming it' (1972: 61). If women living on low incomes were to learn to describe (and help us understand) how they interact with the financial world, they would collectively have to find their own 'language of money'. When we embarked together on the theatre training workshops, we did not know what that language would look like. Despite its dominance, there is a strange silence around personal experiences of money in our society. As SARK, author of woman-centred personal development literature says, 'We are all involved in the same money system, yet we don't share our experiences openly or very often. We lie awake at 3am worrying about bills and have money triumphs alone ... Open dialogues about money are as rare as no credit card debt' (SARK 2002: n.p). Silenced financial experience is difficult to name, but unnamed, it cannot be challenged. However, difficult experiences can be 'storied' in order to make them more manageable; we make sense of them by weaving them into our identities and life stories (Herman 1992, Stanley 1994). Severe or chronic lack of money may not be perceived as a trauma, yet financial crises cause poverty, deprivation and isolation leaving behind feelings of abject failure, shame and hopelessness. We wanted to break the norm and create spaces for money talk, so that women could speak into that silence and name their experiences in ways that were true to them.

Positing Critical Questions

Despite its hidden aspects, learning about money is inherently boring for most people – we hoped theatre would spice it up. Not surprisingly, our willing participants were more energised by life challenges than the topic of finances. We would have been happy to work with mundane stories of confusing bank statements, overdue electricity bills or missed Centrelink[6] payments, but the world of household finances remained stubbornly vague, and in order to avoid imposing an existing discourse we deliberately did not provide clues. The theatre training began with asking critical questions as prompts, but the obvious question, 'What financial information do you need?' meant little to the participants, so we settled on 'What are your experiences with money and with the money system?' This question was then posed in myriad ways such as 'Who is in this struggle with you?', 'Where might it be taking place?' and 'What reality were we inside of?'

Shaping Generative Themes

Three five-minute plays, each ending in a moment of crisis, grew out of the training workshops. The theatre facilitator's skill was to uncover, identify and shape the generative themes. The women's discussions identified the following themes around their financial experiences: being silenced (friendships being contaminated by asking for 'too much' financial help), contradictory (young people can be both financially demanding and protective of a parent in crisis), energising (how exploited migrant women can get support), emotionally powerful (the family dynamics produced when one family member has more financial power than

---

6 Centrelink is an Australian government agency that delivers a range of social security payments and services.

others), and change the women's ways of seeing (the child's eye view of a mother juggling financial demands). If the participants' unique biographies and months of community-based training could be summed up, it would be with this reflection from a woman who after finishing a workshop said, 'I felt we did well. We had to dig deep. I brought things up I have suppressed for so long. It's amazing you can draw on these horrible experiences and it can really help.'

Through the theatre method, participants presented riveting responses to our question about financial information. They told us what the smokescreen of financial literacy was hiding: as Xris put it, 'issues of poverty, isolation and internalisation of an identity as a low income person shape your choices and sense of self-worth.'

Performing the Stories

The participants were asked if they were willing to go on to the performance phase. Ten women agreed to continue, attending additional workshops to shape the plays further. A 'rehearsal' performance was held for the participants' friends and family with subsequent performances scheduled in eight locations. Performance venues included a community house, a support service for marginalised women, a community information centre, a secondary college, and the Macquarie Bank performance described at this chapter's beginning. The research included recording statements made by spect-actors in the facilitated discussions that were part of the performances. This provided valuable evidence that learning extended to the spect-actors as well as participants.

The play 'Family Finances' portrayed financial inequalities between genders, generations and ethnicities. One performance included spect-actors from a domestic violence service who, in the facilitated discussions, related to the relative powerlessness of the character playing a woman without her own income. This is a section of the play's discussion:

- 'How do you get out of a traditional relationship once you are in it?'
- 'You need power at the very beginning of the relationship'.
- 'Being in the paid workforce you get more status'.
- 'The truth is those most powerful in the world are those with money'.

Another play, 'Out of her Depth', portrayed a mother unable to pay the bills and unable to ask for help. The spect-actors of one performance included women who had lived on society's fringes; discussion after the play was about getting help from services, 'I am from the country and I don't socialise and for years and years, I didn't know you could go to churches and get a couple of bags of food. You don't know where to look for something if you don't know it exists', and 'Centrelink have social workers who are helpful but it's actually getting to them …'

This led to a discussion about not knowing about 'no fee' bank accounts for people on income support, 'I only just found out after years. They don't advertise it. How are you supposed to know? It should be bank policy that they let you know. I resent that they send me glossy brochures and don't advertise this.' This is learning grounded in lived experience. It also points sharply to the mechanisms of marginalisation and the policy changes that could make a difference.

As part of the research audience members were also surveyed afterwards on the personal impact of the performance. People spoke of having their awareness raised about the struggles others have had just to get by. It was not the 'financial literacy' instruction that people expected: it was community art touching deeper levels of human experience. As one audience member explained:

'It was great being in the audience. You can really feel a position that every person in the audience is coming to and everyone around them changes too. My insight today was, you change one word or action in a conflict and it can be more positive. A thousand people have told me that but until I saw it being acted out I never believed it.'

It seems that rather than providing *information*, at the lower end of the hierarchy of knowledge, being an audience spect-actor created higher order *understanding*: 'I got a better sense, not that I don't already logically know [it], but I connected more with the experience of it.'

Layers of Learning

A published research report, *Money, Dignity and Inclusion,* has documented this research/training project and produced two frameworks (Landvogt 2008). The first describes the four requirements for financial capability: an adequate income; a fair financial market (regulation); having a personal financial buffer (such as assets) and being financially educated. The second framework is for a four stage community development approach to financial education, shown in Table 4.2.

The report was important for our policy work, but the theatre process opened minds in other ways. For the participants it was not only training about financial matters that was important but learning to advocate for themselves. It was the movement from learning to advocacy that enabled us to make sense of this process, as both an action research process and as a community-based training experience. The movement to collective action is essential, including taking self-advocacy to other stages where people that are more powerful usually 'perform' their policy, research or marketing. For example, the *Money, Dignity and Inclusion* report was launched at Parliament House, shared at an Australian Banking summit and captured on DVD for use with community groups. By putting their experiences on the broader 'stage' of policy the value of the participants' voices became indisputable.

Table 4.2   Community development approach to financial education

	Stage 1	Stage 2	Stage 3	Stage 4
Task	Identify key information points	Facilitate dialogue	Use income maximisation framework	Access resources
Principles	Proactive approach to accessibility; target life transitions and crises	Adult learning, women's learning, and empowerment methods	Information and support regarding: financial information, rights and responsibilities, entitlements, minimising costs, future protection, and getting assistance	Use relevant topics and materials based on participants' self-identified needs
Outcome	Engagement	Participation	Empowerment	Knowledge and skills

In participating, the women overcame barriers, such as mental health crises, homelessness, chronic illness, speaking little English, extended family needs and insecure employment. They did this for themselves, to support each other and importantly, to educate community, government and researchers about their lives and what should change. This is an expression of active citizenship for people who have few opportunities to contribute publicly (Lister 1997). One participant summed it up, 'For me financial issues have always been there. Because I was so worried about my financial problem I never thought it would interest other people. Now I see that expressing this is an opportunity for *others* as well.'

Conclusion

Placing community-based training at the heart of this research project opened up many possibilities: the chance for us to directly hear the voices of those who are usually silenced, and for them to be empowered in the knowledge that they have been heard. In turn, our research offered the community-based training process the somewhat unusual chance to extensively document and share its learnings (Sloman 2011). bell hooks speaks of stepping over the line of what a teacher is expected to teach into a more exciting and unscripted pedagogy (Burke 2004). Community-based training steps over that line. This research also steps into the unknown, guided by curiosity and the quest for emancipation. Like hooks, we searched out the political in the personal, using the art form of theatre as the circuit breaker of habituated researcher-researched, teacher-learner positions.

For Freire (1982) '[t]he task is not to teach people to think – they can already think; but to exchange our ways of thinking with each other and look together for better ways ..' (cited in Frankenstein 2005). We did not set out to teach but rather to learn together through a creative collaboration. Participants unearthed their individual knowledge; created new collective stories with the power to reflect marginalised experiences; and developed plays which critically analysed systemic oppressions, such as lack of affordable housing, financial inequality in the home, and the social stigma of financial dependence. Asked what their experiences with money indicated about what is needed, participants did not nominate financial literacy training. Instead, their insights led us to propose an alternative to the dominant financial education approach, that is, a community-based training process based in dialogic learning and structural change.

References

ANZ and Nielsen, A.C. 2005. *ANZ Survey of Adult Financial Literacy in Australia.* North Melbourne: The Social Research Centre.

Boal, A. 1979. *Theatre of the Oppressed.* London: Pluto Press.

Boal, A. 1992. *Games for Actors and Non-Actors.* London: Routledge.

Burke, B. 2004. bell hooks on education, [Online: *the encyclopedia of informal education*]. Available at: http://www.infed.org/thinkers/hooks.htm [Accessed: 23 July 2011].

Butler, S. and Wintram, C. 1991. *Feminist Groupwork.* London: Sage.

Financial Literacy Foundation and DBM Consultants. 2007. *Financial Literacy: Australians Understanding Money.* Canberra: Australian Government.

Frankenstein, M. 2005. *Reading the World with Maths: Goals for a Critical Mathematical Literacy Curriculum* [Online]. Available at: http://www.nottingham.ac.uk/csme/meas/papers/frankenstein.html [accessed: 23 July 2011].

Freire, P. 1972. *Pedagogy of the Oppressed.* London: Penguin.

Good Shepherd Youth & Family Service. 2011. *Who we are* [Online]. Available at: http://www.goodshepvic.org.au/page/22/who-we-are [accessed: 14 October 2011].

Herman, J. 1992. *Trauma and Recovery: From Domestic Abuse to Political Terror.* London: Harper Collins.

Kempson, E. 2006. *Measuring Financial Capability: An Exploratory Study.* Bristol: Personal Finance Research Centre: University of Bristol.

Landvogt, K. 2006. *Critical Financial Capability: Developing an Alternative Model.* Victoria: Good Shepherd Youth & Family Service.

Landvogt, K. 2008. *Money, Dignity and Inclusion: The Role of Financial Capability.* Victoria: Good Shepherd Youth & Family Service.

Lister, R. 1997. *Citizenship: Feminist Perspectives.* London: Macmillan.

National Consumer Credit Protection Amendment Act 2010 (no. 9), Canberra: Australian Government.

OECD. 2005. *Recommendation on Principles and Good Practices for Financial Education and Awareness.* Paris: OECD Public Affairs Division.

Paterson, D. 1995. *Theatre of the Oppressed Workshops* [Online]. Available at: www.wwcd.org/action/Boal.html [accessed: 22 July 2011].

SARK. 2002. *Prosperity Pie: How to Relax About Money and Everything Else.* New York: Fireside.

Sen, A. 1999. *Development as Freedom.* New York: Anchor Books.

Sloman, A. 2011. Using participatory theatre in international community development, *Community Development Journal Advance Access.* doi:10.1093/cdj/bsq059

Stanley, L. 1994. The knowing because experiencing subject: Narratives, lives and autobiographies, in *Knowing the Difference: Feminist Perspectives in Epistemology*, edited by K. Lennon and M. Whitford. London: Routledge, pp.132–48.

Third-Way Theatre. [Online: Third-Way Theatre Act '4' Change]. Available at: http://www.thirdwaytheatre.org/ [accessed: 23 July 2011].

WIRE. (2007). Women's Financial Literacy Research Report. [Online]. Available at http://www.wire.org.au/wp-content/uploads/2010/08/WomensFinancial LiteracyResearchReport2007.pdf [accessed: 14 October 2011].

Chapter 5

Learning to Strategise, Strategising to Learn: Reflection on Pedagogy of the Change Agency in Australia

James Whelan and Sam La Rocca
with Holly Hammond, Jason MacLeod and Pru Gell

Without a coherent and shared strategy, many community activists and organisers throw everything they have at a problem, hoping that a stream of diverse tactics will somehow generate the required political momentum to create change. Our popular education work, with social movement groups during the 1990s, indicated that many activists were unsure how to develop a campaign strategy to focus their efforts and create tangible change. In fact, in some campaigning organisations, strategy is viewed as voodoo science and its practitioners as sorcerers who guide campaigns through magic or intuition.

Members of our activist education collective became curious about how community groups develop campaign strategies through inclusive, empowering and 'savvy' processes. Our 'Strategising for Change' (SfC) action research project began in 2003 when we collaborated with Philadelphia-based Training for Change (TfC) to lead a series of campaign strategy workshops around Australia. Since then, we have led strategy workshops, mentored campaigners and developed resources that are now being used by many social change groups. In the process, we have learnt not only about campaign strategy but also about political education and conscientisation.

This chapter traces our action learning about campaign strategy and examines how the SfC project helped define our individual and shared pedagogy. The Change Agency (tCA) is an informal collective of educators and facilitators whose work with social movement organisations and activists includes education and training, facilitation, action research and mentoring. In recent years, our collective has supported community-based groups in their quests for social and environmental justice throughout Australia and the Asia-Pacific region.

Some members of our collective were engaged in facilitation and educational work with social movements for many years before we connected. During 2002–2004, James and Sam managed a series of informal workshops where experienced campaigners and educators shared their knowledge. Increasingly, though, the collective took an active role in this educational work.

December 2004 presented a turning point when a good friend gave James and Sam a stern 'practice-what-you-preach' talking to. Our friend's advice made sense. If we believed that our work could build power in social movements and that it was about fostering a long-term shift toward a learning culture, we needed to approach it in a more planned, supported and strategic way. We needed to think bigger and focus our energies.

Our initial response was to reflect on the work we had been doing. Who had participated in our workshops? What were their experiences and priorities? We had been strong on evaluation, so we had summaries of participants' feedback and debrief notes from every workshop. A few things were clear. Firstly, there was strong demand. We could always fill a room, people offered lots of suggestions for future workshops, and were applying their new skills and confidence with positive results. Secondly, we observed that activists love tactics to the extent that we sometimes fail to ensure that they build on each other, that they are connected to our objectives or add value to other movement activities. The consequence can be that campaigns are basically a sequence of isolated activities and action, none of which can realistically be expected to bring about the desired changes.

We also observed that many activists are curiously reluctant to break complex social and environmental injustices down into smaller pieces that are more workable. Perhaps people fear they will undermine the integrity of their political ideology or forget that everything connects to everything else. Or, that focusing on one (potentially winnable) political objective might communicate the sense that other objectives are less important. This reluctance to focus on specific, tangible changes can lead to activist 'shopping lists' of impossible demands.

Some activists seem to think that being strategic means compromising our integrity and principles. Others think that being strategic is the domain of heroic lone-ranger campaigners who have been initiated into the dark science of strategy and that the rest of us have very little to offer.

Instead of focusing on bite-sized solutions, activists tend to discuss problems in rich, elaborate and paralysing detail. Sometimes these discussions are accompanied by solutions thinking, occasionally by contextual and ideological analysis. But, most often they are saturated with more talk about tactics. What can we do? What have we done? What might we do? But, what are we trying to achieve? Few activists seemed to be talking about outcomes or social change processes.

Perhaps these conversations about strategy were not happening because there was not a shared language: phrases with shared meaning to describe different concepts and theories of change. Looking around, members of our collective observed few group strategising processes or tools.

One question about strategy that we turned to was, 'Who or what needs to change?' Within our collective, we were conscious of the tensions between personal, community and political change and how that influences what we choose to educate about (or what we think people need to learn), and how we facilitate, train, educate and counsel. Each member of our group approached these potentially competing priorities of personal growth, group, community health and structural change differently. Some argued that people's need to do work on themselves can be a distraction from political action. Others responded that personal change is integral to becoming an effective activist. To overcome this duality, we discussed how personal change can lead to political change (or campaigning with a more explicitly structural change focus) and how achieving change through politically strategic campaigns can lead to personal growth. We saw that these beliefs influenced *what* we choose to teach or educate about, the content of the work we design and lead, *how* we choose to facilitate and *what we value* as learning outcomes and teachable moments.

Based on these observations, we committed ourselves to strengthening the capacity of grassroots movements to strategise more frequently and more effectively, and to win. Sam's research into factors that influence participation in social movements showed that people need to feel like they can make a difference before they will even get involved in activism, and that they are most likely to develop a long-term commitment to social change if they feel like they are making a difference (La Rocca 2004). This insight fed our desire to develop a shared language around strategy so activists could have deeper and more strategic conversations about their campaigns.

We also wanted to use experiential learning processes to do this, so we began a discussion with George Lakey, founder of TfC in Philadelphia. George and his team were widely respected for their highly participatory approach to strategy and movement building. Like our collective, TfC's pedagogy is informed by theorists including Paulo Freire, bell hooks and Ira Shor, as well as social movement education initiatives including the Highlander Center in Tennessee and the Movement for a New Society. We hoped that their tools and processes would complement our analysis and extend our pedagogy. These discussions led to an initial series of workshops in most Australian state capitals.

In May and June 2005, we led a series of public workshops with TfC's Daniel Hunter. The project was conceived as a series of five to ten workshops for a team of three educator-facilitators, but it rapidly grew. Ultimately, SfC became a focus for a number of our collective members over several years and created opportunities to work in unexpected places with diverse groups – large international non-government organisations, environmentalists in Fiji, Treaty activists in Aotearoa (New Zealand), pro-independence activists in Melanesia, queer and transgendered activists in East Africa.

We seriously underestimated the demand for strategising for change support. When we started to promote strategising workshops and resources to help community activists and organisers, the response was enthusiastic. Perhaps because the project was an action research project and promised to share the resulting resources online, people saw how their movements might benefit and many generously contributed great resources and ideas. We expanded our website to include a new 'strategy' section and it quickly became our most frequently visited page. Each month, thousands of visitors download the 'do-it-yourself' strategising resources and process guides for facilitators.

Through this and other activist education projects during 2005–2010, we built relationships with other educators and grew into a collective. The work was intense. We worked directly with up to one thousand activists and dozens of social movement groups each year throughout Australia and internationally. Our collective was strongly committed to co-facilitation, including focused preparation, collaboration and reflection. This created opportunities to regularly challenge each other (and ourselves!) but until now we have not written about these learnings. To write this chapter we each reflected on a learning 'moment', each of which is presented in the remainder of this chapter. Our reflections reveal quite different, but related, insights.

Sam: The Personal in Activist Education

Catherine Delahunty of the Kotare Trust in Aotearoa once said to me that in social change 'the effectiveness of our actions relies on the quality of our relationships'. I have sat with that ever since, wondering if the quality of our relationships also relies on the effectiveness of our actions.

Our collective has enjoyed a strong connection with Kotare Trust. During their 2006 summer school for activist educators, I presented tCA's interpretation of Steve Chase's (2000) five dimensions of activist learning. Drawing on Steve's framework, we argued that effective activists need to learn: (i) 'content' knowledge about problems and solutions; (ii) big picture political strategy and analysis; (iii) social action skills (media, organising, direct action); (iv) organisational development and maintenance; and (v) personal growth and transformation. I added that tCA was less interested in the fifth – 'middle class navel-gazing that distracts people from the real work'. Kay Robin, an inspiring Māori educator and facilitator challenged me. She was not convinced that that is how it works, especially in a Māori context where people need to start with personal growth and transformation, deal with trauma and get in touch with culture, before they focus on working for structural change.

Daniel Hunter expressed a similar belief: people need to transform their personal blocks to be good strategists. This is probably what some community development practitioners would say about working with people and groups on the margins. Until people believe things can change and that they can be a part of making that change, they cannot engage in activist work.

But, what if people have an experience of winning? Young people organising to get their neglected public pool fixed in a remote Aboriginal community; farmers protecting prime agricultural land from coal seam gas extraction; landowners in the Pacific developing community-owned small-scale logging enterprises that replace large-scale multinational corporations; networks of wine growers and horse breeders stopping a coal mine; Papuan students overturning the law that inhibits freedom of speech; Ugandan *kuchus* successfully convincing authorities to include lesbian, gay, bisexual, transgender/transexual, intersex and queer

(LGBTIQ) perspectives in HIV education. I believe if people have an experience of winning, of organising effectively and achieving a goal that their sense of self grows and commitments deepen.

While working on the SfC project I have been struck by the number of people who cannot imagine winning. Sometimes it is because we do not believe we have what it takes to win something even small.

When facilitating strategy work with our Melanesian friends, Jason MacLeod and I encountered personal and cultural beliefs that deny activists their own true power; leading them to believe that someone else is the expert, that the expert can solve the problem and that the campaign cannot be won without external influence. It is true that international solidarity will be one part of a solution to many conflicts on indigenous lands, but the real experts are those working for peace and justice in their own context.

We have used TfC's 'people-sized strategy board game' to draw out this sense of personal power. One time, as per usual, we invited people to write down all the critical challenges they felt were holding the movement back from winning. We told everyone that we had invited a panel of experts to solve their challenges and provide important advice to enable the movement to win. We asked people to leave the room so we could prepare it for the experts' arrival (meaning we could tape lines on the floor of the big hall for the people-sized board). The excitement was brewing. People were so energised by the idea that, finally, experts were coming to provide the answers they needed to move their campaign forward. Some waited at the entrance for the experts' taxi to arrive. We called people in and started playing the game. Small teams were presented with their own challenges to solve, one by one, in order to move through the board game and reach the finish line, which symbolised 'freedom'.

The exercise served its purpose: participants generated creative solutions to the challenges they had identified and, when the 'experts' turned out to be a fiction, they realised that they were the experts they had been waiting for. The challenges were not insurmountable and the wisdom and courage to overcome each challenge already resided within the group. By taking responsibility for asking and answering the questions that held them back, participants acknowledged their own potential.

I believe the new experiences we have of ourselves and our group 'inside' a learning environment influences how we are 'outside' of it. My experience facilitating strategic processes deepens my appreciation for the role that personal growth and development can have in strategic thinking and effective action. And, at the same time I remain committed to finding ways to use effective action to build strong relationships.

Holly: Education and Facilitation in Pursuit of Effective Strategy

In our activist education work we have grappled with the relationship between education and facilitation. A key difference between facilitation and education seems to me to be the objectives of a gathering we are invited to guide, such as a workshop or meeting. Is it about gaining clarity about an idea, reaching a decision, developing a plan, or ensuring that discussions are engaging and fair? Or is it about learning, understanding, developing a skill, and leaving at the end of the day with a sounder knowledge of something?

Educational workshops generally include many aspects of facilitation. Experiential education is highly facilitative, drawing on the wisdom and experience in the room. Our experiential activities often give individuals and groups valuable time for reflection and for planning their campaigns. At the end of a workshop, which has been primarily focused on learning, participants often leave with a clearer idea of key aspects of their campaign. Butchers paper listing tactics or preliminary stakeholder analysis are kept and taken to the next meeting to inform deliberations.

Likewise, when we have been called on to facilitate campaign planning we have tended to do a significant amount of education about strategy concepts and tools. In order for people to develop a critical path analysis for their campaign they need to understand the tool and its purpose. We frequently use a campaign strategy chart as a workshop resource and aid to planning. The chart sets out the key elements of campaign strategy, such as vision, objectives, stakeholders and tactics. Using this chart effectively for planning requires education about what the different terms mean and how they relate to the overall plan. Education about the value of campaign strategy tends to be a precondition for effective planning.

The relationship between education and facilitation surfaced in an interesting way with one of our project partners. We worked with this organisation over a number of years providing education and mentoring about campaign strategy, activist education and facilitation. The organisation has a strong 'do it yourself' ethos. Once we had introduced them to our curriculum and pedagogy they jumped into developing strategy for their campaigns and running their own workshops.

On one occasion, Sam and I were asked to facilitate the development of one of their campaign strategies at their annual planning meeting held over a number of days. At the previous year's meeting some of their participants had facilitated planning for the same campaign. The result had been an extremely ambitious plan which they were unable to make much progress on. We recognised that their level of understanding of campaign strategy had contributed to this outcome – the group needed more education in order to plan effectively. This informed our workshop design and engagement with the group. In a sense our objective went beyond the development of a clear campaign plan to the kind of experience we wanted participants to have in their campaigning in the year ahead. We hoped for the kind of experience that would build confidence and commitment to campaigning, and hopefully allow the organisation to chalk up some wins and grow in power and influence. We envisaged educational outcomes both within the workshop and the campaign.

Both education and facilitation have been valuable approaches in increasing the capacity of groups to campaign effectively. Our educational work has led to a shared understanding of campaign strategy concepts and tools. Education about past campaigns, successful and otherwise, helps campaigners to envisage the consequence of different strategic choices. Facilitation enables reflection and valuable group conversations about values, vision, and the way forward. The SfC project involved weaving both together, and placing the emphasis on each at different times, depending on the needs and objectives of the group.

Jason: A Simple Exercise Opens up a Transformative Conversation

The lexicon of strategy is sometimes confusing for people. There is a complex language to learn: vision; goals; objectives strategy; and tactics, just to start. One of the objectives of SfC was to help develop a shared language and understanding of strategy amongst the activists and movements we work with. To do this we used a number of tools including the 'Blanket Game', an adventure-based learning (ABL) exercise we adapted from our friends at TfC.

The activity is quite simple. First of all, we generate a list of all the terms people associate with strategising. Then we place a blanket on the floor and ask the group to stand on the blanket. The more crowded, the more challenging! We explain the challenge: the group needs to turn the blanket over without anyone stepping off, even momentarily. If anyone leaves the blanket, the group needs to start again, but they can take as long as they need. After the group completes the task successfully, facilitators guide a reflection on the task. What was the vision in this challenge? What was your group's objective? What tactics did you consider and use? What was your strategy? Sometimes we draw on examples from the group or the broader world to make a stronger connection between the exercise and real life challenges.

The beauty of ABL activities like the Blanket Game is the way group dynamics – and at times movement dynamics – show up. This happened in a workshop we facilitated with a group of young indigenous women in the Pacific. All the participants were active in campaigns for self-determination, economic justice and equality. The women were not only excluded from fully participating in the social, economic and political life of their home countries, they were also subjected to repression from local security forces because of their work for justice. In addition they were struggling against a range of cultural values that justified domestic and sexual violence against them. After failing to complete the Blanket Game several times, the women finally succeeded. They exploded with delight, which gave way to spontaneous singing and dancing.

James Whelan and I, and two local women we were co-facilitating with observed that the women had imposed an additional rule upon themselves: that they could not use their hands to help turn the blanket over. One or two of the participants insisted that they were not allowed to use their hands; as a result the rule was readily accepted by the whole group. So, although the women eventually succeeded in completing the exercise, they made it *much* more difficult for themselves.

An animated debrief opened up. Once the group had discussed the different meanings of the words on the list they had generated at the beginning of the exercise, we shared our noticing that the participants had not used their hands during the exercise.

At first there was disbelief, then shock and mixed feelings when they realised they had limited themselves in this way. Some members of the group were angry with the facilitators for not correcting them. We supported the group to express their rage at the effect of oppression and violence on their lives. After talking for a while about the external obstacles that prevented the women from realising their goals for justice and peace, we then asked them if there any other obstacles that they imposed on themselves; obstacles that constrain their ability to achieve their goals in similar ways to the 'rule' they imposed about not using their hands during the exercise.

What followed was a moment of awakening: a deeper conversation about the nature of oppression and power. Using their experience during the Blanket Game as a reference point, we invited the women to talk about how oppression can be internalised, accepting and replicating the oppressive beliefs held by the mainstream (in this case men) about particular marginalised groups (in this case women). We asked the women how these internalised beliefs functioned to constrain their power to create change. The women discussed the ways they limit their own power, the 'rules' they impose on themselves, the false beliefs men and others hold about them that they unconsciously accept – that they are stupid, weak, dirty or not fully human (and other oppressive attitudes), the times when they do not speak up, the reasons why they do not work together, as well as the structural nature of oppression on their own lives. At this point, just as we teetered on the edge of a problem-saturated conversation, we moved the dialogue to the ways women maximise their power – how they awaken their power-from-within, nurture power-with, experiment with power-to, and undermine power-over. In the spirit of emergent design, it was a discussion that determined the next session on power, which then became a whole day's focus of the workshop.

The conversation about internalised oppression that flowed from this debrief was unplanned. This dynamic is not unique to these particular women. Many activists – men, as well as women – and especially oppressed (or other-than-mainstream) groups limit their power through internalising the oppressive (and false) beliefs that dominant groups in society hold about them, making the challenges they face even harder. It is an exciting moment when these self-imposed constraints are recognised for what they are, revealing the inner architecture of oppression and the ways different groups collude with their own oppression. For an educator, these are times when people grow before you and the world sparkles with possibilities of a brighter future. It was also a reminder to me that even the most basic and routine of exercises can yield opportunities for transformative learning.

Pru: A Mandate to Strategise and the Power of Stories

One hat that I wear is being an activist educator and another is being an organiser whose work is focused on Indigenous peoples' rights. When I work as an activist educator with other organisers who focus on Indigenous rights activism, I wear both of these hats at the same time. As a non-Indigenous person whichever hat I am wearing, I aspire to be an ally for Indigenous peoples. When it comes to Indigenous rights activism, I have observed that some people are not always as strategic and effective as they would like to be. For the non-Indigenous people involved in this work it may be that they do not feel that they have a mandate to do their organising work. If people are uncertain of their mandate, it can affect how confident they are undertaking this work. While this is not a reason for inaction, it may mean that they do not have the necessary robust conversations and hence avoid tackling difficult questions. This makes it difficult to develop winning campaign strategies.

One night during a three-day 'Treaty Worker' gathering James and I were co-facilitating at the Whaiora Marae in Auckland, we were treated to a wonderful story. Storytelling is often a key part of the agenda for our activist educator peers in Aotearoa. The storyteller was Mitzi Nairn, a seasoned anti-racism activist and Treaty Educator in Aotearoa and an elder in the Treaty justice movement. During her story, Mitzi described a dinner table conversation, which took place one night in 1975, when she and her Pākehā (non-Māori), Māori rights solidarity and anti-racist activists acknowledged that they had been given a clear mandate from Māori activist groups who they worked alongside. They had been told, 'We will assert our rights and sovereignty. Work in your communities to prepare Pākehā to support, not block, us as we empower ourselves.'

Here I had an 'ah-ha' moment for two reasons. Firstly, as an activist educator I was sharply reminded of the powerful role that storytelling, and specifically intergenerational storytelling, can play in our activist education work. Mitzi's story reminded me that stories are an accessible way to pass on learnings and highlight skills and lessons. Secondly, I heard wisdom in Mitzi's reflections about her movement's mandate. It was clear that she and other anti-racist campaigners in Aotearoa felt confident they had a mandate from the Māori people to campaign for Treaty justice. Without this clear sense of mandate, it can be difficult to facilitate robust strategising, to challenge the assumption that people can achieve their political objectives through habitual tactics, and to introduce tCA's strategising tools.

I have incorporated storytelling into my 'Indigenous People and Others Working Together Respectfully and Effectively for Indigenous Rights' workshops where people plan their inter-cultural work. Before Mitzi's sharing, I rarely allocated much workshop time for storytelling. But, her story enabled such rich sharing and activist learning. It was important, too, that the workshop format, facilitation and timeframe were fluid. I think that sometimes as a facilitator I hold the reins tightly, managing the time and possibly the 'container' (sense of connectedness and focus in the group) too tightly. This led me to think about the benefits of emergent design and going with the energy of a group.

Experiencing Mitzi's storytelling also made me reflect on the different facilitation approaches in tCA's team. I thought about one of our tCA facilitators who has a less hands-on facilitation style than me, who is comfortable with emergent design and more likely than me to give lots of time to storytelling.

My insights during Mitzi's sharing highlighted the importance of asking Indigenous and non-Indigenous organisers to share stories that draw out the learnings from their work. For example, during workshops I ask participants to respond to some questions in their storytelling such as, 'What has supported your inter-cultural activist work?' and 'What would it take to work together in a way that is genuinely respectful and mutually useful?' As a popular educator, I have learnt that personal experience *is* the curriculum and the source of theory.

James: Peer Learning Through Co-facilitation

At the end of each day, our debriefing discussions were focused and energetic. We talked through what went well, identified how we might do things differently next time, provided 'critical friend' feedback to each other and shared other observations. What 'ah-ha' moments or other useful learning outcomes were evident? How were participants relating to the concepts and tools? To each other? To us as facilitators? Were there moments that really 'went live'? What 'learning edges' were people encountering? Were they outside their comfort zones? Had we made the right decisions about content, sequence and timing? How would we do things different next time?

These discussions were priceless. By challenging each other, inviting critique and remaining open to the possibility of other, potentially better ways to approach our educational objectives, we learnt actively and the workshops improved quickly. We did not always agree! There were moments when deep differences were apparent in our beliefs – differences that reflected our diverse political beliefs, educational philosophies and convictions about individual and group learning. At times, I felt very challenged. In fact, there were moments of conflict and tears in our facilitation team, as well as moments of inspiration, celebration and learning.

After a Brisbane workshop, I asked Daniel to talk about one session he had led that had left me puzzled. During the workshop an outspoken member of the group had challenged him, 'This exercise isn't well thought through. I can think of a better way to approach this strategising process.' In response, other members of the group either contributed their ideas or encouraged each other to engage in Daniel's suggested process. Daniel, meantime, withdrew to his seat and appeared to disengage. I watched the interaction, confused. Why did he disengage? Why not explain, justify and assert the process? I recalled that when we prepared the workshop, we had designed this session to introduce a strategising process we considered important for people to learn and apply. Instead they had quite a different discussion. Daniel explained to me that in that moment in the workshop he had deliberately chosen to let the group storm. Becoming a group, breaking free of the domination of the educator-facilitator and exercising agency were important to their learning.

A year later, I was working with members of a student union when I remembered Daniel's choice. Workshop participants were reluctant to agree to each other's suggested campaign objectives and tactics. It became clear that there were significant underlying tensions and a struggle around power and leadership within their group. Putting our workshop agenda aside, we invited people to name some of these dynamics and speak about how they were affecting the union's political work. Some group members were comfortable in this discussion. Others resisted at first, arguing that it was not the workshop they had signed up for. They acknowledged, though, that working on how they functioned as a group – making decisions, listening to each other, sharing responsibility and learning – was necessary before they could achieve their political objectives (or even to agree on them!).

These moments in the project convinced me of the value of co-facilitation and team teaching. We learnt so much from each other! Our structured approach to collaborative preparation and debriefing helped me realise the interconnectedness of the various dimensions of activist learning. Reflecting on the complex interactions we had encountered during workshops, I saw that learning to work together and exercise agency are just as important as learning to strategise, and these learning dimensions cannot be neatly separated. The means and the ends are equally important.

Conclusion

These five reflections reflect the diversity of experiences, ideas and orientations within our small collective. They also point to shared insights that have guided our development as individual educators and as a team with a clear philosophy (or praxis).

Firstly, we have discovered that learning can become a central and valued element of the culture in social change groups, organisations and movements. The expressions 'learning organisation' and 'learning culture' are common in organisational management literature, but social movement groups typically value 'doing' over learning. Who has time for mentoring or workshops when there is a planet to save? The SfC project helped open a space where reflection and sharing, analysing and theorising, incorporating new information and planning for action – the stages in the experiential learning cycle – are valued and valid exercises. Over the years, we have observed significant cultural change in some groups where learning now receives more attention than previously. We also work to embody a learning culture within our collective through intentional peer learning and reflective processes.

Secondly, we have learnt that empowering activist education involves several learning dimensions that cannot be neatly separated. It is useful to have a framework (like Steve Chase's five dimensions), but that does not mean we can neatly delineate the forms of learning to address in a workshop. As people learn and practice strategising skills, they may simultaneously find opportunities for applied political analysis or explore how to work more effectively in groups. The SfC project would not have realised its potential if we had categorised our work simply as instrumental training and focused exclusively on imparting practical and replicable skills. Instead, we drew equally on the traditions of popular education: valuing and eliciting participants' experiences; teaching people new skills; helping create learning groups; encouraging active and respectful listening; and facilitating groups' development.

Thirdly, we have learnt about the centrality of personal experience in activist education. Some of the richest learning has emerged from discussions and exercises that were not part of carefully designed workshop plans and curriculum. This is not to imply that preparation is unnecessary, or that there is no merit in a deliberately designed series of exercises. But, educators cannot anticipate the wisdom that participants bring with them, the urgent challenges they face and problems they are passionately committed to solving. Through story-telling, participatory and experiential processes, and bringing our own experiences and interests to our educational work, we can honour and harness the power of personal experience.

The Strategising for Change project provided rich learning opportunities for our collective. We have learnt about our pedagogy and priorities, the movements we work with, our co-facilitators and ourselves. In some ways, the project has come to a close in a formal sense, but we will all continue to grow as a result of this deep learning.

References

Chase, S. 2000. *The Education and Training Needs of Environmental Advocates and Organizers*. New York: University of New England. Unpublished.

La Rocca, S. 2004. *Making a Difference: The Factors that Influence Participation in Grassroots Environmental Activism in Australia*. Honours thesis, Australian School of Environmental Studies, Griffith University. [Online]. Available at: http://www.thechangeagency.org/_dbase_upl/LaRocca_honours_final.pdf [accessed 21 December 2011].

Chapter 6

A Re-imagined Identity: Building a Movement in Brisbane for the Practice of Social Role Valorization

Lynda Shevellar, Jane Sherwin and Gregory Mackay

It's 2002. I've just come out of a committee meeting of our local organising group (Brisbane), where there has been a great deal of conversation about our community education experience. Despite rich discussion, one topic is not progressing: the movement from theory to action. It is as if we're stuck. We want to honour the people this work is truly for; we want to honour the tradition of our educational efforts; yet we also know that we have a collective role in change and we could be doing more to make inroads.

I struggle to articulate my concerns. I see a very limited repertoire of training options: a theory event taught in a top-down didactic manner, along with a highly structured practicum event. People seem to get a great deal from the training. But I'm left wondering whether there is real transformation when they return to their everyday lives after the training experience.

Undoubtedly, a few do go on to make a difference. Where they are successful in making change is in situations where they have supportive others, particularly supervisors, or where they have linked with others of a similar mind. I suspect what we use to prepare people for action is not adequate. It is sometimes stimulating, interesting and engaging but ultimately it is theory. I'm left wondering how can we rethink what we do and how we do it as a collective? (Community organisation member and educator)

Introduction

The three authors of this chapter belong to a global community of educators, practitioners and change agents committed to transforming the lives of people who experience social devaluation through the use of Social Role Valorization (SRV) theory (Wolfensberger 1983, Kendrick 1994, Wolfensberger 1998, Race 1999, Wolfensberger and Thomas 2007). Over the past three decades, we have witnessed the capacity of this theory to transform the lives of those who are vulnerable, as well as those families, allies and workers who stand alongside them. We have been part of efforts to apply the theory to assist the closure of institutions and to support people with a devalued status moving into community life. We have glimpsed the possibilities for larger scale transformation through the adoption of key SRV principles within legislation, such as the Australian Commonwealth Disability Services Act (1986) and subsequent state government legislation. Despite these achievements, we remain frustrated in our educational efforts, conscious that the potential of this work has not yet been realised.

This chapter tells the story of an ongoing struggle to build on the transformative experience of individuals. In doing so, our hope is to create a collective of people who use SRV theory in their thinking and in their practice to create community change. However, as the opening story portrays, there are tensions for participants and for facilitators. Through this chapter, we seek to name these points of tension in our practice. In doing so, we explore the kinds of ideas offered by community-based education and training that could offer a way forward for us.

The opening vignette is offered by one of the authors who is a member of a local organising group committed to the dissemination of SRV theory. This group is unfunded and has no paid staff, an active membership of about forty people, and a broader network of one thousand people. Its primary purpose is to foster the learning and application of SRV theory.

The opening vignette also captures the first tension that we hold. We want to acknowledge the importance and usefulness of SRV theory, but also point to frustrations in our education and training experiences. In writing this chapter, we have felt the tension between community action and professional development. For although SRV education and training explicitly values the ordinary everyday lives of community members, the focus is typically on human service delivery and evaluation. We are also conscious of the characteristics of workshop participants. People with disabilities, their families, and members of other marginalised groups are encouraged and even actively supported to attend events. Yet the majority of the participants also carry an organisational role as providers and/or recipients of human services: roles which they struggle to set aside during the learning experience.

In addition, the SRV training material is 'owned' by the Training Institute for Human Service Planning, Leadership and Change Agentry (Training Institute) at Syracuse University in New York State. This ownership exists through intellectual property rights and copyright. More importantly, it sanctions what, by whom and in what ways the material can be taught. This echoes the role of professional associations and licensing bodies that perform gatekeeping functions in other fields, such as in psychology, social work, medicine, accountancy, law and so forth.

While the educational strategies tend to be conservative in nature, the politics of the theory are inherently radical: there is an ultimate agenda of social change and the theory has been adopted by progressive social movements within the disability sector.

This leads us to conclude that SRV theory continues to have great relevance and is highly potent in shaping conscious and helpful responses to the needs of people who are marginalised. At the same time, the personal experience of exposure to the theory in itself has limited potency to transform social systems and communities. As change agents, community educators and organisers it is this tension we struggle to hold and which now invites us deeper into our story.

Reflecting on the Participant Experience

> It is October 2002 and the third day of a three-day SRV theory training event. I was warned that the content would be intellectually rigorous and that the days would be long and tough, but I hadn't appreciated how emotionally exhausting it would be. I spent the first day deeply touched by the stories of pain and rejection. This led me to reflect on my own contribution to these experiences of marginalised people, especially at the hands of the service system. Then yesterday I felt so energised. I wanted to run out and begin making a difference in the world. But now on our final day together, I'm just feeling overwhelmed. I want to talk about how I can make a difference, but there doesn't seem to be any space. The examples they show us seem clear; yet I know my own context is complicated. I want someone to help me think it through. And I'm feeling so helpless. I know when I go back to my workplace I will be on my own. I also know I will never see the world the same way again. How do I help others to see what I can now so clearly see? (SRV participant)

These participant reflections capture the experience of SRV training from the learner's perspective. It demonstrates the capacity of SRV training events to lead to critical insight and awareness. At the same time, it points to some of the limitations and challenges of present educational endeavours.

Articulated by German-American psychologist and philosopher Wolf Wolfensberger (1983, 1998), SRV is founded on a deep understanding of social devaluation. It explains why it is that people with certain characteristics are more likely to be perceived negatively, and responded to in ways that equate to marginalisation and social exclusion. It provides means for citizens and organisations to respond to this societal dynamic. Key to this understanding is the theme of consciousness-raising, which echoes Paulo Freire's ideas of conscientisation (1970).

It is hoped that during the SRV training experiences, participants will strengthen their own personal identification with the plight of people who have a devalued status. This speaks to some of the central tenets of adult education, including the valuing of personal experience, the desire for direct problem solving and a learning incentive driven by the individual (Knowles 1980). John O'Brien (1999) refers to the challenge that participants eventually face as they are confronted by the realities of social devaluation: To what extent are they willing to confront the possibility that some of their own practices could be contributing to devaluation and further wounding, and to what extent are they prepared to say, about their own practices, 'STOP!'?

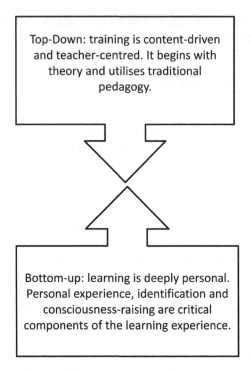

Figure 6.1   The tension of bottom-up and top-down

At the same time, the educational format ignores contemporary normative adult learning principles and instead applies a top-down approach to learning. In Australia, the dissemination of SRV has been primarily through workshops (these consist of two-, three- and four-day versions with varying degrees of intensity and depth). Any one of these three workshops is a prerequisite for the practicum workshop, called PASSING (Wolfensberger and Thomas 2007).

Within the theory workshops, the learning is structured and the pace is pre-determined in a schedule of topics. There is sequencing of learning that requires people to be exposed to the theory first and then to do the practicum, so that they receive the 'coherent logic and integrity of the overarching theory and its assumptions' (Thomas 1999: 363). There is little use of experiential, elicitive, dialogical or participative learning. Instead, the main learning method is lecture format. Learners sit in a classroom setting. PowerPoint slides are used extensively throughout, providing a visual summary of the key learning points as well as illustrations. The lecture format suggests that participants are blank slates and that the role of the educator, understood to be a teacher, is to fill that slate. It clearly represents the orthodox pedagogy model discussed in Chapter 2 of this book, with a focus upon gaining facts, and a largely passive role for the learner. This has led to criticism of the theory, even though what more rightly needs to be targeted is how it is taught.

The practicum involves visits to human services, time spent with service recipients, and then reflection. The points of reference are an SRV-based evaluation tool and the citizens' knowledge of typical societal dynamics.

This melding of consciousness-raising with a classroom approach to learning provides another point of tension in the SRV training experience. We see this as the top-down and bottom-up tension, as depicted in Figure 6.1. This same dynamic is evident in the relationships among the SRV trainers, the Australasian accreditation body and the official Training Institute at Syracuse University. In our multiple roles, we have felt this tension: wanting to honour the extraordinary body of work developed over decades by colleagues we hold in high admiration, and knowing the value of the safeguards around the content, but wondering how more flexible processes might be integrated into the SRV Theory events. The next section will elaborate on this.

Reflecting on the Trainer Experience

> I am in the role of Senior Trainer, in the midst of teaching SRV theory to 25 people. This is hosted by the local organising group and I am conscious of wanting to do a good teaching job for the sake of the participants and the local group, but especially for the vulnerable marginalised people whose devaluation this theory goes some way to addressing.
>
> By my side are the trappings of teaching and learning: the teaching script and PowerPoint slides. I am conscious that I am carrying on the tradition of how this theory has been taught across Australia, Great Britain, Scandinavia, America, Canada, and New Zealand for at least the past two decades. In the margins of the scripts are my examples that I'll use to try to bring the script to life. I will try to take a stance that is confident, yet engaging. I feel the pressure of needing to cover a lot of material in a relatively short period of time, and of adhering to the slides and script. I feel for the participants and hope that they will be supportive of the co-presenter trying to teach a complex theory using the teaching script for the first time.
>
> I am wondering about how much people really benefit when exposed to having to learn this way. Are these training modes sufficient in themselves? What else is necessary so that people can apply what they learn? Learning about and trying to apply SRV has a huge impact on the lives of participants; but what else is required to ensure effective application of the theory to real life situations? (SRV Trainer)

Two concerns are flagged in this SRV Trainer reflection: the safeguards around content and process, and what happens to people's learning after the classroom experience.

The issue of protecting the authenticity of the content is a central concern for the Training Institute and is both a strength and a weakness in the education process. Firstly, the content is managed in a way that results in controlling the process. Scripts and presentation materials (handouts and PowerPoint slides) are provided for the three- and four-day workshops. These scripts were developed at the Training Institute by Wolf Wolfensberger and colleagues. There are yet more rigorous and systematic requirements before one can be considered competent to teach SRV at an accredited level. Only those who have reached accredited Senior Trainer status have access to a full set of scripts. Those who are co-presenting receive copies only of the sections that they are presenting. Part of the negotiations in receiving the scripts is that they are not to be disseminated to unauthorised people. A national safeguarding and accreditation body has responsibility for this safeguard.

Secondly, the processes that are used to teach the material are also highly structured: this results in standardised workshops. Australia and New Zealand have adopted this mode in imitation of the American scene (Thomas 1999). It is expected that the presenters follow the scripts, which use a didactic form of teaching. These measures all work to ensure consistency in the material that is presented, and to minimise the likelihood of marginally related or inaccurate concepts being taught under the banner of SRV.

Thus, what we see is a theory embedded in a rich and rigorous framework, based upon empirical work, taught by people with a strong social justice agenda. It addresses matters of profound significance, it speaks to timeless realities in the lives of marginalised people, it puts forward strategies that are potentially highly beneficial and it continues to be relevant despite being developed in the early 1980s (Kendrick 1994).

However, in reflecting upon our experiences we also see four clear patterns of concern. Firstly, there is a disconnection between people's transformational experiences within the classroom and the application of this theory in people's daily lives. Despite positive individual feedback about the SRV event, what we observe is rapid dispersal of learners after they leave the classroom. Few go on to undertake the practicum and even fewer remain connected to the network of people implementing change. On returning to their lives and to their workplaces, not many participants continue the important conversations to keep the learning alive.

Secondly, there is a lack of take-up of SRV theory by those in leadership roles in organisations, and therefore there is a widespread lack of application of the theory. An exception to this was noted by Millier (1999). Currently there exist progressive responses to the needs of people with disabilities in Australia with leaders who have been informed by SRV. At the same time, we know that these pockets of good practice constitute the exception rather than the rule.

Thirdly, an emphasis upon the content over the learning has meant an emphasis upon theory over application. While the theory has been safeguarded, its application has not. Thus, we observe many odd and even damaging practices within disability, mental health and aged care settings – some of which are even undertaken in the name of SRV. Many participants nod sagely at the theory, yet remain unable to influence the culture and practice of their own service settings.

Fourthly, in the mid-1980s and 1990s, there occurred widespread closure of institutions arising from the application of SRV theory. This happened throughout Australia and sat alongside similar international liberation efforts. Yet even now, as we write this chapter, new oppressive policies and initiatives are being rolled out across Queensland, Australia – so far with minimal resistance.

These paradoxes and contradictions lead us to pursue a deeper analysis of the dissemination of SRV. In the next section we ask what might it take to move from our current approach to something that fosters not only application of the theory, but that also fosters social change through collective transformation?

Our Analysis of the Dissemination of SRV: Moving Towards a Transformational Agenda

As authors, we have used the 'spiral model' of transformational learning, depicted in Figure 6.2, as a way of reflecting on the dissemination of SRV theory and to assist us to develop an analysis, enabling a way forward. This model is used extensively in popular education, that is, education that facilitates critical examination of one's own social world. It provides a step-by-step process that helps individuals and groups to identify areas of common concern and to address these issues by working together. It suggests that the starting place is the experience of the participants: to reflect on those experiences and then seek patterns.

SRV theory is grounded in experience, but unlike many other education and training experiences, the focus within SRV theory is on the 'other'. By this we mean that the *subjects* of the training – people who are marginalised – become the *objects* of the training. This is to a certain extent impossible to avoid as the training focuses on the lives of many people who cannot participate or even be present due to the complex nature of their disabilities, severity of illness or their incarceration within institutions. Instead, the participants are those members of the community who stand alongside them as allies, companions, family members, advocates, supporters, volunteers and paid workers who can, and do act with them and on their behalf. In understanding the experience of devaluation, SRV training therefore does not start from the experience of the participants, rather it starts from the experience of those people who participants stand alongside. Within SRV training events, the voices of the people who are most marginalised are uplifted; but the consequence is that the actual training participants sometimes feel excluded and silenced. We wonder what it might be like to instead start with the experiences of those who are present, to invite them to tell their stories of what they have seen and how they have responded.

The second step involves looking for patterns. SRV theory does identify patterns; however, these are largely predetermined. Participants have limited

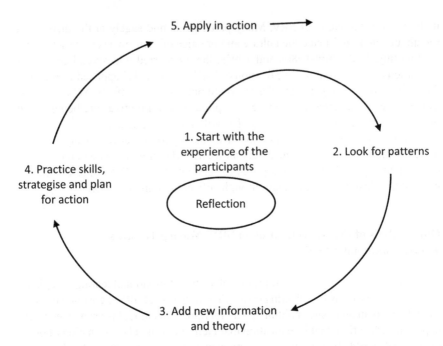

Source: Used with permission from Rick Arnold, Bev Burke, Carl James, D'Arcy Martin, and Barb Thomas. *Educating for a change*, Toronto: Between the Lines, 1991.

Figure 6.2   The spiral model

opportunity to engage with their own contribution to devaluation and valuation, and to recognise such patterns for themselves.

The third step within the spiral learning model is the inclusion of theory and information. Within SRV training, the theory is the starting place rather than an addition to participants' own reflections. If we invert the SRV training process and start with people's experiences, then SRV theory might provide answers to some of the questions people are asking, rather than impose an agenda.

The fourth step in the spiral model is to connect with the new knowledge, practice skills and to strategise and plan for action. Certainly, this occurs within SRV training with exposure to the use of positively valued social roles, such as employee, student, neighbour, as a key strategy for overcoming devaluation. However, this occurs purely within the classroom. Outside of the classroom, we imagine creating the space for discussions on applying SRV theory within the context of people's lives, and the creation of safe and nurturing spaces for ongoing story-telling, reflection, and a deepening of understanding.

Finally, the fifth step calls for applying strategies in action. The spiral model invites us to understand this as an open space in which our local education approaches might gain momentum.

What the spiral model of learning assists us to conceptualise is the opportunity for a re-imagined learning space. This analysis has also illuminated three things needed to create a future whereby individuals and organisations utilise SRV as a means of countering oppression and furthering better lives for people with a devalued status. We need to strengthen the personal transformation of individuals, connect these individuals to each other, and have ways of supporting their efforts. This is explored in the next section.

Reflecting on the Experience of the Community Organisation Member and Educator

Jump forward a decade to 2012: the local group is now a vehicle for fostering and supporting people in their efforts at social change. Participants feel like they are part of something, that their efforts matter and, very importantly, that their experiences, successful or not, are highly relevant and indeed welcomed by the broader group.

We've moved beyond our initial ideas of expanding the way we engage in training. Those ideas were restricted to bringing people to learn more, and in more flexible ways, yet somehow fell short of meeting the real needs of participants.

Now we ask people to join us so that we are together on a journey of learning to use the theory of SRV. We ask members to lead with their reflections on how they use SRV theory, on how they struggle in doing so, and what they've learnt to do differently. The journey continues to be interesting: we frequently struggle to ensure we are learning together rather than mis-learning together.

The next steps are becoming obvious. We need to find ways to introduce experiential, elicitive, dialogical and participative learning in a range of forums. This could be done while still teaching the theory, so as not to lose the depth and richness of the theory itself. This part of the journey speaks to the challenge of exploring through relationships and working out alternatives to what has seemingly been set in stone. We know we can travel this road because our colleagues across Australia and the world share in a deep-seated desire to see people who are marginalised moving to living full and generous lives. (Community organisation member and educator)

In the past ten years, we have spent time individually and collectively, informally and formally, with people who were affected by what they had learnt and who had shown enthusiasm to go further but who had also struggled to do so. We listened and we changed or added events and approaches where we could. And it is making a difference.

Firstly, we added small and quite informal supportive events such as breakfasts and discussion evenings to build our sense of a learning community. Breakfasts have been a great opportunity for people to come together socially, be reminded of who else is in this effort, and to have a facilitated discussion about a topical event through the SRV lens. Exploring technical aspects in using the theory is a significant part of the discussion evenings. Importantly, these are framed over supper, and with both formal presentation and facilitated elicitive discussion.

Then there have been attempts to respond to people's desire to be assisted in the application of this theory. We have come together in a large group in a short session to explore, discuss, plan, reflect and act, and then commit to a smaller group based on interest and/or geography. After that, participants go about their everyday lives trying to implement the actions from the workshop. Then, a few weeks later, each small group meets. Here they share critique and ideas for improvements on their efforts.

The final piece of the puzzle has happened over the past year or two. In an effort to build our learning community, we are exploring how we might best describe our identity. We are increasingly operating in the manner of a community of practice. We are drawn to Etienne Wenger's definition of communities of practice as groups of people who share a concern or a passion for something they do and learn how to do it better as they interact regularly (Wenger, McDermott and Snyder 2002).

We see how the identity of a community of practice can more deliberately assist our reformation. For the vast majority of people learning about SRV, there has been no peer support for individuals whatever their role. In contrast, in a community of practice, it is not only the way in which content is taught that is important, but also the peer supports that exist for people in their efforts to apply what they have learnt.

In undertaking this transition, we are observing our own shifts from students and trainers to thinking about our roles as learners and facilitators. In terms of SRV training it means shifting from a teacher focused orientation to a learner focused one. It means shifting the centrality of hosting an SRV theory event to seeing the theory event as one learning experience in a range of transformational opportunities. It does not mean changing the way theory might be presented, however, it does mean rethinking its place within a broader cycle – and community – of learning.

A Re-imagined Way of Being

This reflection confirms the importance of a re-imagined space. This is presented in Figure 6.3, using what Tony Kelly and Sandra Sewell refer to as a trialectic, or a 'logic of wholeness' (1988: 22) to more firmly evolve and embed a community-based training approach. Trialectic logic helps move us out of binary dilemmas, such as the top-down and bottom-up tension observed in the opening of this chapter. According to Kelly and Sewell, a trialectic establishes a third factor as a point of focus. In doing so, new insights into social realities can emerge and new ways to problem-solve develop.

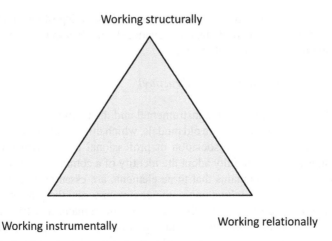

Figure 6.3   A new trialectic for transformation

The three focal points are: *working instrumentally* in which work is task-focused; *working relationally*, which requires paying attention to the interpersonal level, that is, building the bonds of trust and reciprocity, generosity and goodwill; and *working structurally*, which means creating an identity and structure that hold these two elements together and facilitates each. The following reflects how the organising group is evolving to work in these three interrelated areas.

Working Instrumentally (Task-focused)

The local organising group has had a long and successful history in organising training events where the focus has been on marketing, organising venues and equipment, providing materials, and liaising with the trainer.

However, more recently, the local group has played a role in creating a new accredited event that better matches the participant learning needs and integrates greater discussion. The local group has also hosted additional events that have a learning function, but equally importantly have the function of bringing people together in an informal setting.

Working Relationally (Interpersonal)

In response to the issue of individuals disconnecting from the wider group after training and becoming isolated from any movement for change, the local group considers people will do better when they are connected to others of a similar mind and engaged in similar efforts. People know each other in a variety of contexts and come together in multiple ways. This is typical of how communities operate. People know each other through SRV events, through work roles and through citizen roles. This is now reflected in the group's informal gatherings where there are attempts to create conversations, share an understanding of the challenges we all face, explore what it would take to advance the application of SRV, and make real change in community and services.

Working Structurally (Identity and Structure)

To hold the tension between the instrumental and the relational we needed a new structure: to move away from the old models, which might include being a training organisation, incorporated association or professional body – and for the local organising group to more fully adopt the identity of a community of practice.

Etienne Wenger maintains that three elements are essential to the identity of a community of practice: the domain, the community, and the practice. Applying this framework, we identify the first element, our domain, as SRV theory. The second element, our community, is made up of people who engage in discussions and share information. They are thought of in three 'layers': the committee of management who work both instrumentally and relationally with each other, then friends and others who participate in the informal gatherings as well as in the formal events, and finally those who engage peripherally through the formal events and then watch and learn from afar. The third element, the practice, supports devalued individuals to have better lives and, in particular, valued roles, while appreciating vulnerability and potential.

Conclusion

As stated in this chapter, the movement to support people moving into the community depends on increasing knowledge and personal transformation, as well as *collective* transformation and action – best understood within a radical community-based education and training tradition. It is extremely helpful to have such a useful and elegant theory, however, we need to do more than hold events and teach the theory. We need to engage participants in ways that will most enable learning and that will foster application of the theory in action. In doing this, we need to avoid group-think ignorance and foster critical examination of one's own actions. We need to keep in mind the higher order goal; that our work is about changing the social conditions surrounding marginalised people. Different teaching and learning processes will be insufficient in themselves. It is asserted that working in more relational ways are also essential, an intention best captured by Margaret Wheatley and Deborah Frieze who say,

> Despite current ads and slogans, the world doesn't change one person at a time. It changes as networks of relationships form among people who discover they share a common cause and vision of what's possible. This is good news for those of intent on changing the world and creating a positive future. Rather than worry about critical mass, our work is to foster critical connections. We don't need to

convince large numbers of people to change; instead, we connect with kindred spirits. Through these relationships, we will develop the new knowledge, practices, courage and commitment that lead to broad-based change. (2006: 1)

References

Arnold, R., Burke. B., James. C., Martin. D. and Thomas. B. 1991. *Educating for a Change*. Toronto: Between the Lines.

Freire, P. 1970. *Pedagogy of the Oppressed*. New York: Continuum.

Freire, P. 2006. *Pedagogy of the Oppressed*. 30th Anniversary Edition. New York: Continuum.

Kelly, A. and Sewell, S. 1988. *With Head, Heart and Hand: Dimensions of Community Building*. 4th Edition. Bowen Hills: Boolarong.

Kendrick, M. 1994. Some reasons why social role valorization is important. *The International Social Role Valorization Journal*, 1(1), 14–19.

Knowles, M.S. 1980. *The Modern Practice of Adult Education: From Pedagogy to Andragogy*. New Jersey: Prentice Hall.

Millier, P. 1999. Normalization and social role valorization in Australia and New Zealand, in *A Quarter-Century of Normalization and Social Role Valorization: Evolution and Impact*, edited by R.J. Flynn and R.A. Lemay. Ottawa: University of Ottawa Press, 447–54.

O'Brien, J. 1999. Education in applying the principle of normalization as a factor in the practical arts of improving services for people with disabilities, in *A Quarter-Century of Normalization and Social Role Valorization: Evolution and Impact*, edited by R.J. Flynn and R.A. Lemay. Ottawa: University of Ottawa Press, 385–92.

Race, D.G. 1999. *Social Role Valorization and the English Experience*. London: Whiting and Birch.

Thomas, S. 1999. Historical background and evolution of normalization-related and social role valorization-related training, in *A Quarter-Century of Normalization and Social Role Valorization: Evolution and Impact*, edited by R.J. Flynn and R.A. Lemay. Ottawa: University of Ottawa Press, 353–74.

Wenger, E., McDermott, R. and Snyder, W. 2002. *Cultivating Communities of Practice: A Guide to Managing Knowledge*. Boston: Harvard Business School Press.

Wheatley, M. and Frieze, D. 2006. *Using Emergence to Take Social Innovation to Scale*. [Online: The Berkana Institute]. Available at: http://www.margaretwheatley.com/articles/using-emergence.pdf [accessed: 18 July 2011].

Wolfensberger, W. 1983. Social role valorization: A proposed new term for the principle of normalisation. *Mental Retardation*, 21(6), 234–9.

Wolfensberger, W. 1998. *A Brief Introduction to Social Role Valorization: A High-Order Concept for Addressing the Plight of Societally Devalued People, and for Structuring Human Services*. 3rd Edition. Syracuse, New York: Training

Institute for Human Service Planning Leadership and Change Agentry, Syracuse University.

Wolfensberger, W. and Thomas, S. 2007. *PASSING: A Tool for Analyzing Service Quality According to Social Role Valorization Criteria. Ratings Manual.* 3rd Revised Edition. Syracuse, New York: Training Institute for Human Service Planning Leadership and Change Agentry, Syracuse University.

Chapter 7

Building Community Leadership from the Inside Out: The Story of the Building Better Communities Training Course in South East Queensland

Howard Buckley

Introduction

In Australia, we often hear the phrase 'community has broken down'. This notion that things are not as they should be in our modern communities has driven a number of responses by governments, non-government organisations and individuals, all seeking remedies that tinker with varying pieces of the puzzle. The varied responses are usually underpinned by assumptions that change can be wrought by doing things *for* or *to* the community. This has shaped generations of people in Australian society into expecting that change is something done to them or for them, thus propagating passive participation in civic and community life.

The 'Building Better Communities' (BBC) training course was established by Community Praxis Co-op to counter this dominant mode of thinking. We wanted to promote the idea of community building as a process rather than an outcome. We saw our task not so much as attempting to *build community* but rather to *create spaces* where community can be built. One way to create such spaces and to enable community members to shift from passive citizenship to active leadership is to initiate community leadership training. This chapter tells the story of our training experiences, and our efforts to support this shift.

The Building Better Communities Community Leadership Training Course

Community Praxis Co-op is a workers' co-operative that provides the collaborative infrastructure for enabling members to earn an income by forming self-managed teams for project, consultancy and training work. The Co-op seeks out and responds to work opportunities that contribute towards building more peaceful, just and sustainable communities. In 1999 Community Praxis Cooperative was contacted by Caboolture Shire Council, in South East Queensland, Australia with a specific request.

The Council had brought together fifteen human service workers to consider the vexing question of how community development (CD) could be advanced in the Shire. What made this discussion interesting was that the focus was not limited to 'let's employ a CD worker' but rather 'how do we create space for community to be nurtured (particularly in new neighbourhoods)?' These conversations led to some members of Community Praxis Co-op being asked to develop and deliver a twenty-hour community leadership training course in a newly formed, rapidly-growing suburb with minimal social infrastructure, where many of its residents were not connected with each other. An extract from Community Praxis' *A Guide to Good Practice* (2003: 6) reveals the seeds of the course that were planted on that day:

> People shared their experiences of community and what they thought were the key ingredients to building safe, healthy neighbourhoods. A common theme emerged around the notion that there were some values and skills that were underlying principles to building community, and that if people could learn and practice these skills this would enhance the building of community in their neighbourhood.

We named this engagement with values and skills 'community leadership training'.

Community leadership training, in its very essence, aims not only to get people to act as leaders, but to instil a capacity to think like leaders. Community leadership training, understood in this way, becomes a far richer experience than merely skills development or adopting a systematic 'how to' manual. It is a process of bringing people together to re-imagine the world another way, to understand the constraints that hold us back, and to collectively mobilise ourselves into action through shared learning. Community-based training and education, understood as a process to achieve this, provides an effective model for delivering community leadership courses.

The first course evolved from the experience two Co-op members had in running a community orientation course in inner city Brisbane[1], Queensland. It was a huge success and led to numerous courses being funded across the Shire over the following five years. Since then the BBC training (as it became known) has been delivered over eighty times throughout communities in South East Queensland. It has become a well-regarded and effective mechanism for mobilising people to enhance their connections and actions in their local communities.

An essential part of the mandate in developing the BBC course was that it could bring a diverse group of people together from disparate backgrounds, support processes of group formation, and then inspire and mobilise the group to collective action. A classroom style, agenda-based training method would not be able to achieve this. The course required that Community Praxis co-op create a training framework that: was experiential for participants to learn new

---

1   See the chapter by Dave Andrews in this book, which gives an account of this inner-city training.

skills; utilised an elicitive training style to ensure that the learning was rooted and grounded in the context of participant's lives; and focused on mobilising for social action. In this framework the trainers would play the roles of facilitator and provocateur more so than teacher.

In this context community leadership training that utilises such a community-based education and training framework becomes a transformational learning exercise with three clear foci:

- *To communicate knowledge to enhance understanding of the processes required to create the spaces where community is built.* This requires bringing together diverse people and groups with an expectation to think differently. It is the paradigm shift work that becomes the core of the training. It is an exercise in challenging prevailing attitudes, behaviours and ideas. Sometimes we have to 'unlearn' before we can learn.
- *To form a safe, connected group that germinates social mobilisation.* The foundation characteristic of building healthy communities is that people are safe and feel safe (Andrews 1996). Likewise, in a training setting, creating a safe space for participants that enables them to share their stories and experiences creates a connectivity that becomes the fertile ground for experimentation and the basis for sustainable action.
- *To equip participants with technical and practical skills that will increase their level of confidence to be an agent for change.* It is essential that the core of the training work remains focused on training participants, as well as educating them. The logic here is to move participants to act, not to merely contemplate what they might do. As Westoby and Shevellar point out earlier in this book, the difference between education and training becomes very clear when participants are expected to 'do' or 'action' the learning in their lives.

The role of training community leaders in this way becomes both exciting and challenging. The trainers take responsibility for guiding the delivery of a course the outcomes of which will be determined by the engagement and willingness of participants to learn new material and skills, and to experiment with this learning in connection with others.

About Building Better Communities Training

The BBC Course is a twenty-hour course that seeks to mobilise participants by developing their confidence, skills and connections to create the kind of community that they would like to live in. The course typically provides an opportunity for up to fifteen participants who have a connection to a locality or to a homogeneous group (such as a group of young people in a school setting) who want to make a difference in that community.

The course uses extensive storytelling as the means for generating discussion and introducing topics, so there is an expectation that participants need to be open to listening to others and have a willingness to share their own stories. The sharing of stories becomes one of the key factors in building a safe, trusting environment upon which a sense of community is built in the group. The creation of this safe space allows a deepening of the connections between participants as they discover where their stories meld and enables the germination and cultivation of collective ideas. The trainers' consciously use the course materials and topic discussions to tease out and nurture relationship building throughout the course. The material is always presented in the context of someone's story, thus grounding the learning and giving it a very real and achievable dimension. However, opportunities for this to occur also happen outside the formal training moments. Community Praxis has designed the course around the sharing of meals together, a key strategy that becomes the soul of each course. Rachel Remen sums up this way of working beautifully when she says:

> Everybody is a story. When I was a child, people sat around kitchen tables and told their stories. We don't do that so much anymore. Sitting around the table telling stories is not just passing time. It is the way the wisdom gets passed along (1996: xxv).

The trainers will also use their own stories of community building experiences, often relating their own struggles, in an attempt to create a space in the group where it is safe for participants to share their painful or confronting stories. This acts as a leveller and helps break down the 'my story is not really worth sharing' syndrome. The use of this strategy also requires the trainers to become vulnerable to the group.

The BBC course is based on adult learning principles, which means the trainers acknowledge that all participants bring skills, knowledge and experience to contribute and the trainers' key role is to create a participatory learning environment. As in all group processes the way discussion is facilitated, the time dedicated proportionately to each topic, the mix of deductive and inductive modes of learning, and the careful diverting of those who like to dominate discussion are all key to how successful the training experience will be.

The trainers do not assume a role as experts, but rather enablers – guiding the group through an enjoyable journey together. Obviously, the trainers bring a level of expertise with them, but use this expertise as a gift to the group rather than in an authoritarian role. Unlike in most education institutions the trainers see their role as being present to the participants and accompanying them as they share their experiences.

The course also has to be fun for participants, it needs predominately to be an interactive experience and the training must be gentle. The use of humour is not only useful but a prerequisite in our training style; there is a need to be open and light in demeanour, which helps to dispel the expert tag. If the trainers are not enjoying themselves, there is little chance the participants will enjoy the experience.

The trainers, however, do have roles in assisting participants to take steps forward and will at times use a technique termed the gift of gentling (Kelly forthcoming) which simply means to nudge, prod and carefully help a person make a shift in learning. Westoby and Dowling (2009: 67) define the gentling process as knowing 'when to push people to try something new, to trust the power of the group, to "walk their talk"'. Yet gentling also requires knowing when to back off, letting go of untimely opportunities, giving people a 'break', all essential skills for trainers using the community-based training and education method. One participant in a course summed this up by saying the course helped them take 'half a step outside their comfort zone'.

The Course Content

Three core sessions build the foundation for the course. In the first session, participants explore the kind of community that they would like to live in. This explores peoples' experience of community and the values implicit in our ideal communities. Topics covered in this session include: articulating a vision for community; collectively identifying some key principles that underpin the values for community building; and identifying some characteristics of healthy communities.

In the second session, the difficulties faced in trying to build our ideal communities are unravelled and some positive ways to increase participants' power are considered. Facilitated discussions include: understanding powerlessness and how we experience power; an analysis of social capital in modern society; and exploration of ways to increase our influence in our communities.

In the third session, participants are introduced to a framework for community building, and to a method for connecting with others in the community. Community Praxis Co-op uses a particular community development method (Lathouras 2010), and specific skills are taught that enable participants to connect with individuals to build participatory action groups. Trainers focus on the importance of participatory groups as a vehicle for social mobilisation and participants learn specific skills to build these types of groups in their own contexts. This session is the heart of the training and is considered the most critical session for many participants. In the remaining sessions participants chose topics that will be of most use for them. Examples of elective topics covered in previous courses include: how to motivate people to get involved; dealing with difficult people; planning and sustaining community projects; and effective campaigning and awareness raising. The composition of the group, the level of depth sought on each topic and the number of sessions planned will determine how many elective topics are covered in each course.

Requirements of Course Participants

During each course, participants are encouraged to do something in their community and use the training as an opportunity to reflect on these actions. The rationale for this is that:

> Enabling experiential learning involves more than simply offering opportunities for participants to have experiences as part of a training process. Learning from experience depends upon opportunities to make sense of experiences. The learning is enhanced by reflecting on old and new information and by making connections with the values/knowledge/skills/attitudes of the learner. This process of integration ensures more effective learning for participants and values the experiences of the person as a source of learning for themselves and others (Community Praxis Co-op 2003: 29).

The training's emphasis on experiential learning in action provides participants with the opportunity to experiment with a piece of work that they are currently involved in, a new initiative that they are keen to start, or to simply work on building relationships to enhance their connectedness in their community.

The Building Better Communities Training as an Expression of Transformational Learning

The BBC training starts with a series of exercises that focus participants on their ideal community by tapping into their aspirations and hopes for community building. This starting point shapes the entire training experience and becomes a foundation upon which the whole course is built. Trainers with Community Praxis hold to the perspective that training is about inspiration, not just information; an idea captured by Antoine de Saint-Exupéry who says: 'If you want to build a ship, don't herd people together to collect wood and don't assign them tasks and work, but rather teach them to long for the endless immensity of the sea' (cited in Illback 2010).

In other words, training is an opportunity to touch a chord with participants to arouse an enthusiasm to re-imagine their world, to discuss possibilities, spark new ideas, and embrace hope. The genuine creation of such a space gives participants the freedom to engage in the 'what it could be like...'. Emerson reflects: 'Though we travel the world over to find the beautiful, we must carry it with us, or we find it not' (1990: 107).

The BBC training has also been described as discovering ourselves in relationship with others. While we are clear that the training is not a series of group therapy sessions, nor is it used to counsel individuals, it is apparent that many people carry personal baggage and so when a group forms we can inadvertently create a 'collective unclaimed baggage depot'. In such situations, the trainers must be careful not to allow particular individual's needs to dominate or deviate from the core of the training.

However, the fine line between what is personal and what is public usually means that there will be some crossover between those lines as the group determines what it can and cannot deal with. This to-ing and fro-ing in training presents transformational opportunities as someone's personal story/issue becomes the catalyst for unravelling a public concern. There are few moments in training stronger than when a participant has shared in a moment of vulnerability, and the group embraces that moment – not in judgement or suspicion – but in compassion and solidarity to shift the matter from the personal realm into the public/collective realm. The willingness of the individual to become vulnerable in this instance becomes an opportunity for group transformation. The following story from one BBC course illustrates this:

> Jack (name changed) is an intelligent, well-informed Indigenous man who has considerable knowledge of Indigenous issues, both locally and at the national level. Jack has been misunderstood by other Indigenous people in [the town] and often when this occurs he goes on the attack and then others reject him and his views. The cycle has continued and has left Jack feeling angry and frustrated and the wider Indigenous community poorer for not listening to Jack's wisdom. During the course, Jack came forward with some very blunt attacks (not directed at anyone in the room) about how 'some people' have tried subversively to destroy a local network for their own gain. What Jack had to say was indisputable. In typical fashion, the room fell silent and people wondered if the attacks were directed at them, or even if they weren't, 'What could they do about it?' Gary (name changed) listened to Jack and took on board some of the comments (not personally but in a vicarious manner) and sought to offer some healing for Jack. This was not the cycle that Jack was used to but it provided him with the opportunity to engage rather than withdraw. Gary and Jack talked about the problems; the rest of the group entered the conversation and others felt comfortable about venting their anger too. Gary became more informed of the history of the network and the group gained a greater appreciation for the people involved, Jack experienced some acceptance, others felt this was a safe space to be heard. This was the beginning of our training (Community Praxis Co-op, DFAC, BCC & CSC 2003: 60).

In another course, the group was discussing the topic of resolving conflict peacefully. Stories were emerging from the group about how various participants had dealt with conflict that they had been involved in which was providing useful material for the trainers to elaborate on conflict resolution processes. However, the session was leaning towards technical responses to conflict and seemed to lack some of the more human elements required. At this point one of the quieter members of the group shared a story of her personal involvement in conflict, which became a catalyst for deepening her relationship with her son:

'Ann' had a son, 'Mark', who had recently moved out of home to study at university. After a few months, it became clear that Mark was struggling with his studies and his life generally. Ann suspected that Mark was involved in using drugs and when she asked him about this, he finally admitted to her that he was smoking marijuana. Ann was shocked and very disappointed. She expressed her disappointment to Mark which led to many arguments. The slow, painful breaking down of their relationship was deeply hurtful for Ann who wanted more than anything to maintain a good relationship with Mark. One day during a heated argument Ann asked why Mark was letting marijuana use destroy his life. Mark responded, 'How would you know what marijuana is like, it's okay for you to sit in judgement but you've never tried it.' In a moment of desperation Ann responded, 'Well I'll try it if you'll talk with me so we can build some understanding together.' Mark thought Ann was not being serious but Ann persisted and eventually they sat down and smoked a joint together! This action led to them talking about what was going on in their lives and was a starting point to developing a much healthier and deeper relationship.

When Ann shared her story with the group, you could have heard a pin drop! For some in the group the idea of Ann, the quiet, middle-aged woman who spoke so softly smoking a joint was inconceivable. Then the group broke into raucous laughter as the image filtered through their minds. As the group realised the lengths to which Ann was prepared to go to heal the conflict with her son, a resonance of deep respect and understanding for Ann overflowed from the participants. A truckload of PowerPoint presentations about conflict resolution could not have come close to providing the transformational learning that was unleashed through Ann's emotional and quirky story.

Moments of personal transformation that become seeds for group transformation are not confined to conflict. The BBC courses are rich with examples that reveal a deeper level of learning for participants. Participant feedback conducted as part of the course evaluations reveals people commonly experience a mind shift during the training. Typically, this mind shift is around the notion that community work is not about the participant as an individual but rather it is about the participant's connection with others, which also occurs within a larger set of processes. Many participants have commented on the shared wisdom held by many community workers to 'hold your agenda lightly' as the seeding moment in which this mind shift takes place. One participant stated in a video evaluation, 'I used to focus on the goal as the important thing but now I realise that achieving *my* goal is not necessary as it's about the community connection and what *we* can achieve that is important' (Community Praxis Co-op 2006, original emphasis).

The transformational mind shift does not remain at an individual level. As another participant stated, 'I now feel equipped with a method that can be carefully placed in the various groups that I'm involved in' (Community Praxis Co-op 2006). Her use of the words 'carefully placed' aptly describes the spirit in which the mind shift occurs. It is not a newly found fundamentalism that propels people to proselytise others but a quiet confidence that a method has been discovered that can be enacted thoughtfully in relationship with others.

Building Better Communities Training as a Catalyst for Social Mobilisation

Utilising a community-based education and training method the BBC courses enable social mobilisation to take place in a developmental way that translates to a grassroots, bottom–up approach that is owned by the people, sourced by the people and undertaken by the people. The training, if effective, will engender not only some learning of orthodox community development movements but also the actual movements themselves will take place throughout the training, mirroring real life. Three of these key community development movements in social mobilisation are:

- the movement from 'I' to 'we' – mobilising individuals into participatory groups
- the movement from 'private concerns' to 'public action' – mobilising ideas into collective agreements to act, and
- the movement from 'to' or 'for' people to 'with' or 'amongst' people – mobilising the shift from the service orientation into solidarity with people.

These three movements challenge the dominant service orientation paradigm in modern Australia, which focuses on working *for* people as individuals, with little analysis of the structures of power embedded within those service oriented practices.

Participants in community-based education and training must become informed, not only of facts and details, but also of the myths and poetry that can carry us, inspire us, and lead us to be change agents in a dysfunctional world. Unlike revolution, that replaces one dominant power with another, social transformation is a process of experimentation that inherently understands that we are part of the change that is required. With this in mind, in each BBC training course a short reading[2] is presented as a text for re-imagining how we can connect with people to initiate change in our communities:

> Go to the people
> Live with them, learn from them, love them
> Start with what they know, build with what they have.
> But with the best leaders
> When the work is done, the task is accomplished
> The people will say, 'We have done this ourselves'.

---

2   This passage, commonly used to inspire community workers, is attributed to Lao Tzu, however there are many variations in translation. See for example, Chapter 17, in Le Guin (1997).

Lao Tzu's simple yet profound 'love them' underpins any social mobilisation that seeks lasting change. The great activists and social mobilisers throughout history all have used radical notions of love to mobilise people, from Jesus' 'love your enemies' through to Gandhi's 'there are no enemies'.

It is this notion of understanding how to love people in a training context that cannot be instrumentally manipulated and therefore invites participants to find a deeper level of understanding and experience upon which to hinge learning. There is a danger in participants over-emphasising the emotional aspects of love. However, love understood as responding to people compassionately and considerately can dispel such fears and open hearts and minds to new opportunities for community building. This approach challenges old ways of working that reinforce the status quo, and re-invigorates hope in the fiery furnace of conflict and doldrums of despair.

The Need to Discern Community Interest from Vested Interest

Community-based education and training offers a unique opportunity to explore how we can deal with the systems and people that are operating from a vested interest. The training room can offer a safe space for participants to free themselves of the shackles of frustration that bind us when dealing with these situations. It enables participants to focus upon how to act differently and to re-imagine what can be achieved. A good example of this was observed during our training experiences in a small rural town.

Historically, farmers and businesses had run the town. In recent years a growing number of young families had begun to move into the town, and it had become evident to some course participants that more was needed for this new group of community members. Some of the ideas mooted were establishing youth events, developing a space for family support services and establishing a playgroup. Unfortunately, some conservative 'older people' in the town had resisted this change with the familiar catch-cry 'if they move here they should just adapt'. The participants in the training were disheartened and were almost at the point of giving up due to the resistance to change that they were observing. The training course provided an opportunity for the disappointment to be aired in a supportive, constructive manner and led to developing strategies to engage with some of the more sympathetic 'older' people who could assist in bringing about change. Two years later another BBC course was held in the town, and the reflections on the work of this original group revealed that they had seeded a myriad of responses that are still part of town's social infrastructure today.

The participants could have quite easily given up when resistance occurred but the course enabled them to frame where this resistance was coming from, and to critically reflect on whether their own ideas were based on developing the characteristics of a healthy community and that they were also in the community's interest. This increased understanding and knowledge gave them a stronger resolve to press on and mobilise others to join then. The impact has been to create a lasting impression in that community.

Conclusion

In Australia today the need to create alternative pathways that bring people together to rediscover that yearning for community is paramount. This chapter has described an experiment in community leadership training that seeks to do just that. The BBC training has been able to actualise the idea that change can be seeded by groups of people committed to what Gandhi so poetically phrased as 'experimenting with truth'. As a form of community-based education and training the BBC courses are an expression of working from the inside out as each course is only as effective as the individuals who collectively participate. The more that we understand that individually and collectively we are the social change that is required, the closer we will get to achieving the change we desire.

References

Andrews, D. 1996. *Building a Better World.* New South Wales: Albatross.

Community Praxis Co-op. 2003. *The Delivery of the Community Praxis Co-op Local Community Builders' Training Course – A Guide to Good Practice.* Australia: Community Praxis Co-op.

Community Praxis Co-op. 2006. *Building Community on the Sunshine Coast Project Evaluation DVD.* Maleny: Community Praxis Co-op.

Community Praxis Co-op, DFAC, BCC and CSC. 2003. *Reviving Local Communities: An Evaluation of the Community Leadership Training Project.* Queensland: Community Praxis Co-op.

Emerson, R.W. 1990. Essays XII: Art. Originally published 1841, from *Essays: First and Second Series*. The Library of America Edition. New York: Vintage Books.

Illback, B. 2010. *Presentation at International Youth Mental Health Conference 2010.* 29–30 July, Melbourne Australia.

Kelly, A. forthcoming. *With Love and a Sense of Necessity.*

Lathouras, A. 2010. 'Developmental community work – A method', in C*ommunity Development Practice: Stories, Method and Meaning*, edited by A. Ingamells, A. Lathouras, R. Wiseman, P. Westoby and F. Caniglia. Melbourne: Common Ground Publishing, pp.11–28.

Le Guin, U.K. 1997. *Lao Tzu: Tao Te Ching. A Book About the Way and the Power of the Way.* Boston: Massachusetts, Shambhala Publications.

Mackay, H. 2007. *Advance Australia... Where?* Sydney: Hachette.

Remen, R.N. 2002. *Kitchen Table Wisdom: Stories that Heal.* Sydney: Pan Macmillan.
Westoby, P. and Dowling, G. 2009. *Dialogical Community Development: With Depth, Solidarity and Hospitality.* Brisbane: Tafina Press.

Chapter 8

Training for Transformation: Reflections on *In situ* Community Work Training in Brisbane

Dave Andrews

Introduction

This chapter provides my reflections on *in situ* community work training in Brisbane, Australia. *In situ* community work training is community work training that takes place in a community in which the participants live and work together. These reflections introduce my journey into *in situ* training, and then situate the training within the context of a community network known as the Waiters Union. The chapter reflects on the training philosophy that has shaped my training approach.

The Key Community Contexts in our Life

Home

Most of the community training that my wife, Ange, and I received was from our parents. Our parents not only took people into their hearts – but also into their home. People going through difficult times would stay for a day, a year, or however long they needed. Our parents were examples to us of how we could become people who were not preoccupied with ourselves, but could create a sense of community with others, particularly with those who are marginalised. Their example provided the perfect *in situ*, on-the-job training environment. So, Ange and I have tried to copy our parents, and tried to set a similar example for our children, friends and colleagues.

Dilaram

In 1972, I graduated and married Ange; we flew to Europe and travelled overland to India. In 1973, with the help of some friends met along the way, we set up some communities in India we called *Dilaram,* or 'Houses of the Peaceful Heart'. These communities catered for weary travellers, trekking up and down the Asian hippie trail in search of enlightenment (or a cheap opiate substitute).

Aashiana

In 1975, we left *Dilaram*, which was working mainly with expatriates, to set up *Aashiana* to work solely with local drug addicts. *Aashiana*, literally means 'nest', and we hoped *Aashiana* would be a nest where people as 'wounded birds' could 'mend their broken wings' and 'learn to fly, free, again'. We helped people on the condition that they would help others. The residential rehabilitation community started by *Aashiana* was incorporated as *Sahara*. And, out of *Sahara* emerged *Sharan*, an innovative, community development organisation, staffed mainly by ex-drug addicts from *Sahara*, who were learning to use their understanding of despair to serve communities who knew nothing but despair.

The Waiters Union

In 1985, we returned to West End, Brisbane, Australia, and again with some other key comrades set up an intentional community network that is called the Waiters Union (Andrews and Beazley 2010). This emergent community network of people decided to call themselves the West End 'Waiters Union' because we wanted to be 'waiters' in West End. We did not want set agendas for people. We just wanted to be available, like waiters, to take people's orders, and to do what we could do to help them. We particularly wanted to help to develop a sense of hospitality in the locality, so that all people, especially people who are usually displaced in areas like ours could really begin to feel at home in the community.

All the work we do is *self-directed* and *other-orientated*. A person becomes a part of the Waiters Union, not by jumping through any hoops, but simply by participating in our activities. We believe that people should have the right to shape all the decisions that impact on their lives. Once a person is a part of the Waiters Union, they have the right to shape it. And we believe the best way for us to shape the impact on our lives, individually and collectively, is through the process of consensus. As we work from the bottom-up to empower people, particularly people who are marginalised, we particularly include people who are usually marginalised in the decision-making process of our activities. So we actually work *with* the people that we work *for*, and in so doing, seek to enable the people we work *with*, as partners, to realise their enormous potential.

Through one group, we seek to promote the aspirations of the Indigenous inhabitants of our neighbourhood. Through another group, we seek to support refugees by sponsoring their settlement and the settlement of their families. And through a whole range of groups we seek to relate to the people in our community, who are physically, intellectually, and emotionally disabled – not as clients – but as friends.

None of these things seem that great. However, we constantly encourage one another to remember that true greatness is not in doing big things, but in doing little things with a lot of love over the long haul.

Community Initiatives Resource Association

The Waiters Union has always been a non-formal community network. Over time, we have come to recognise the need for a formal community organisation as an auspice for some of our community activities. Usually groups solve this problem by turning their non-formal community network into a formal community organisation. However, in the move towards such institutionalisation, they lose the very charisma of community. Therefore, we decided that we would not institutionalise our community under any circumstances.

Instead a sub-group of people in the Waiters Union set up a formal organisation as a parallel structure alongside the non-formal network, so that if anyone in the community needed an officially recognised, legally registered auspice[1] for certain activities, they could use the Community Initiatives Resource Association (Westoby, Hope-Simpson and Owen 2009). To make sure this Association only serves as an auspice for the Waiters Union, and does not have the power to co-opt the Waiters Union, it has been designed as a minimalist organisation – with minimal power – apart from its capacity to function as an official, legal auspice for the community.

Since its inception, the Resource Association has provided an auspice for managing community property, providing compulsory public liability insurance and supplying volunteers with the status required by the state. However, by far the Association's greatest role has been to help establish community programmes, which needed legal backing for funding with maximum accountability, but minimal control. The Resource Association has helped establish dozens of community programmes including the Creative Stress Solutions Project, the Inner City Citizens Advocacy Group and Community Praxis Co-op.

In situ Community Work Training Options provided by the Waiters Union

Some time ago, we were asked to set up some training in community work based on our West End experience. Most of the training provided by people in the Waiters Union occurs informally as an integral unpaid part of their ordinary everyday life.

However, a more formal community-based training programme has been developed. These days a training team operates as an initiative under the auspices of the Community Initiatives Resource Association offering seven training options:

---

1   In Australia funding is often only available to community organisations legally structured in particular ways (for example as incorporated associations, companies). An auspicing arrangement is a contract that enables one group to apply for, hold and administer funding on behalf of another.

- We provide an initial introduction to our community work training though one hour Community Work Talks. These talks are preliminary presentations that provide a gentle introduction to our 'compassionate community work training'.
- We provide one-day Community Work Workshops. These workshops are preparatory seminars on the spiritual, personal and relational dynamics of compassionate community work.
- We provide two-week intensive Community Orientation Courses. The course is a grassroots, face-to-face, show-and-tell, do-it-and-discuss-it introduction to compassionate community work. There are a range of inputs from community members involved with Indigenous Australian peoples, refugees and people with disabilities in the neighbourhood, as well as people experimenting with alternative initiatives based on fair trade, inclusion, cooperation, nonviolence and sustainability.
- We provide three-month Community Work Placements. These placements provide an opportunity for people who want an introductory live-in experience of community work in general and compassionate community work with the poor, in particular. It involves living in a supervised community household and being involved in a range of community activities. Mostly university and seminary students looking for community work placements take up this training option.
- We provide six-to-twelve-months Community Work Internships. These internships provide an opportunity for people who want an advanced experience of community work. It involves living in a supervised community household and being involved in a range of community activities. Usually members of the household do not work or study full-time so that they have more time to connect with, and support people and groups in the community.
- Our Compassionate Community Work Course, which is usually delivered over one year, addresses two units of competency from the Australian Community Services Training Package. The first unit focuses on support for community participation. The second unit focuses on support for community leadership. This course is delivered externally throughout Australia in partnership with several tertiary institutions.
- Finally, we run Project Hope for half a day every six weeks. It encourages faith-based community workers to integrate a radical spirituality and community life. Some of its key concerns are: helping participants develop a healthy balance between their inner and outer lives and strengthening congruence between their personal spirituality and their public activities; challenging people to move out of their obsessions with self and into practical others-orientated faith; and encouraging people to think of how they can sustain themselves long term in compassionate community work rather than being crippled by discouragement. Project Hope meetings are characterised by interactions with people around South East Queensland

and Northern New South Wales who share their experience of grappling with the complexities of compassionate community work in their localities.

In situ Community Work Training Philosophy

I hope that any community work training that we do encourages non-formal, transformational, spiritual, experiential, personal, relational, principle-based, and politically committed practices. This section reflects on each of these elements of a training philosophy that I have found useful within my practice.

Formal and Non-formal Training

Formal community development training is usually conducted in an institution. Non-formal community development training is usually conducted in the context of the community itself. Whereas formal community development training tends to be inflexible, with the content for the learners set by the teachers, non-formal community development training tends to be flexible, with content that is set by a community of teachers and learners together.

Most of the community development training I have participated in has been non-formal rather formal, but the formal training that I have participated in informs my non-formal training. The most useful formal community development training I have received was at the Department of Social Work and Social Policy at The University of Queensland, under the guidance of Dr Allan Halladay, who was Head of the Department, and Tony Kelly, who was the Senior Lecturer in Community Development.

When I start to think about the most useful formal community development training that I have provided, I begin to feel more ambivalent. On the one hand, there is no doubt in my mind that the training I did at various TAFE[2] colleges, was of great help to many people; pitched as it was, at a very practical level. On the other hand, I found TAFE colleges the most difficult educational institutions I have ever tried to work with. In each of the three cases where I tried to work with TAFE colleges, the unhealthy culture of the institution adversely affected the healthy quality of the education that we were seeking to deliver.

These experiences only served to reinforce the notion that we needed to find a way to deliver good quality, practical, community development courses outside the formal constraints of the TAFE system. And for us, this has meant developing community development training options for small groups in non-formal *in situ* locations. With community education processes it is best to incorporate flexible

---

2   TAFE stands for Technical and Further Education. It is a publicly funded post-secondary educational organisation in Australia, which provides a range of technical and vocational education and training courses. It is similar to institutions in other countries known as Polytechnics, Vocational Technical Colleges or Community Colleges.

content prepared by practitioners, with the help of experts, rather than by experts themselves. The aim of this approach is to create co-learning communities who will test their learning through action and reflection in the context of ordinary everyday life. Table 8.1 contrasts the two kinds of training.

Table 8.1 Contrasting community development training

Formal community development training	Non-formal community development training
Large groups in formal institutional locations	Small groups in non-formal *in situ* locations
With school education processes	With community education processes
Fixed content, prepared by experts	Flexible content, prepared by practitioners
Teachers teach and learners learn	Facilitators create a co-learning community
Learning tested by summative evaluation	Learning tested by action and reflection

The Spiritual Dimension of Training

My training philosophy is informed by the realisation that our world is in trouble; and religion, which was meant to make things better, but has often made things worse. We do not suffer from the lack of religion, but from the lack of love. Therefore, if we are to have any hope of survival, we need to find a way to be able to care for ourselves and for our world, once again. It is my view that a radical spirituality of compassion is not merely our best hope; it is our only hope. The basis for compassion is empathy. Empathy is the capacity for us to feel how others feel. It is in empathising with people in danger or distress that we can be motivated to refrain from harming them, and perhaps, consider helping them (Goleman 1995: 328–9). Moreover, while most of us might be willing to give intellectual assent in our heads to rediscover our capacity for empathy, it simply will not happen, unless all of us give some emotional affirmation to that intellectual assent in our hearts and make it happen (Macmurray 1968: 28–9).

John Macmurray reflects that the only way we can live, is to live in the real world. And the only way we can live in the real world, is to love the real world. And the only way we can love the real world, is to overcome our fear of the suffering that love in the real world involves. We must not allow our fear of the suffering to take over our lives so that we put all our efforts into building up our defences against the world, thereby alienating ourselves from the very reality we need to relate to. We need to find a faith that can help us overcome our fear of the suffering, so that we can embrace the world as it is, love it, warts and all, and live our lives, with friend and foe alike, to the full. It is my hope that the training we provide would serve as a step along the way for people exploring a spirituality of compassion, empathy and love that is essential for developing 'community'.

Experiential Dimension of Training

Clark (1975: 4–5) argues that, 'there are two essentials for the existence of community: a sense of significance and sense of solidarity. The strength of community within any given group is determined by the degree to which its members experience both a sense of solidarity and a sense of significance within it'. One of my hopes is that any training provided in relation to community would include the opportunity for people to experience this sentiment; the sense of significance and solidarity at the heart of community. I hope they would also experience the training as an opportunity to develop deep mutual respect for one another like, in a healthy extended family. This is far from mere romanticism. Sociologist Luther Smith (1994) identified the primary indicator of community wellbeing as fellowship, which approximates the qualities of a caring family. Part of training would therefore include a nuanced understanding of the idea of community. As Scott Peck asserts:

> If we are going to use the word [community] meaningfully we must restrict it to a group of individuals who have learned how to communicate honestly with each other, whose relationships go deeper than their masks of composure, and who have developed some significant commitment to 'rejoice together, mourn together', and to 'delight in each other, make others' conditions our own.' (1987: 59).

Similarly, Clark in his book *Basic Communities* (1975) says that community is essentially a sentiment which people have about themselves in relation to themselves: a sentiment expressed in action, but still basically a feeling. Such authors remind us that any community-based training process needs to focus on the experiential element of community within the training space.

Personal Dimension of Training

Community development is a personal issue; it begins with us. We all have the ability to choose, but if we want to bring about change then we need to choose to be proactive, rather than reactive. Reactive people are often affected by their physical environment. If the weather is good, they feel good. If it is not, it affects their performance. Proactive people can carry their own weather with them. Whether it rains or shines makes no difference to them. They are value driven; and if their value is to produce good quality work, it is not reliant on the weather conducive or not.

Reactive people are also affected by their social environment, by the 'social weather'. When people treat them well, they feel well; when people do not, they do not function well. Reactive people build their lives around the behaviour of others, empowering other people to control them. Proactive people feel the effects of their social environment, take the 'social weather' into account, and decide how they are going to deal with the conditions. Whether people treat them well or not, they do the best they can. Proactive people build their lives around their own behaviour, developing their power over themselves to exercise increasing control over their responses.

It is only as people become less reactive, and more proactive, that they can actually become more responsible. Stephen Covey, the famous American life coach says:

> 'Look at the word responsibility – 'responseability' – the ability to choose your response. Highly proactive people recognize that responsibility. They do not blame circumstances, conditions, or conditioning for their behavior. Their behavior is a product of their own conscious choice, based on values, rather than a product of their conditions, based on [un-thought through] feeling.' (Covey 1989: 71).

Covey concedes this is very hard to accept especially if we have had years and years of explaining our misery in the name of circumstance. However, until a person can say deeply and honestly, 'I am what I am today because of the choices I made yesterday', that person cannot say, 'I choose otherwise'.

It would be my hope that any training we would provide serves as an opportunity for people to develop greater self-awareness: a capacity to choose a response to the world, and a capacity to change the world proactively.

Relational Dimension of Training

Community development is not only a personal issue it is also a relational issue. Change may start with us, but if it stops with us it will stop altogether. We need to make changes, but others need to make changes too. Unless we all choose to relate to one another proactively, we can never hope to experience a healthy sense of community with one another. Robert Putnam (2000) says that if we are to develop healthy communities then we need to move beyond merely bonding with people who are like-minded people to bridging the gaps between people who do not appear to be like-minded at all. This thinking moves us from community as an ideal, to an experience of community that exists through our relationships with one another.

Community may be worth striving for, but it is not an ideal that can ever be realised over an ideological battle. Community, as previously stated, is essentially 'a sense of significance and sense of solidarity' that comes through developing relationships that are characterised by mutual respect. The loss of mutual respect in relationships strikes a deathblow at the very heart of a community (Smith 1994: 100). Hence, it is vital for us to keep in mind the maxim made famous by Dietrich Bonhoeffer, the anti-Nazi martyr, who said, 'He who loves community destroys community; he who loves the [people] builds community' (cited in Vanier 1992: 35).

It would be my hope that any training provided would serve as an opportunity for people to develop awareness of ourselves as persons-in-relationships, and of our need to move from dependence, through independence, towards interdependence, characterised by developing relationships of mutual respect between people, regardless of culture, class or creed.

Principle-based Dimension of Training

If we are to help people develop the principles required to develop community, then we need to help people not only clarify their values, but also commit themselves to a substantive set of values, without which healthy community development is a complete impossibility. I often reflect on the words of Stephen Covey who argues: 'The principles I am referring to are not esoteric, mysterious, or "religious" ideas. There is not one principle .. that is unique to any specific religion, including my own. These principles are a part of every major enduring religion, as well as enduring social philosophical and ethical systems' (1989: 34). Covey also asserts:

> Principles are guidelines for human conduct that are proven to have enduring, permanent value. They're fundamental. They're essentially unarguable because they are self-evident. One way to quickly grasp the self-evident nature of principles is to simply consider the absurdity of attempting to live an effective life based on their opposites. (Covey 1989: 34)

Probably the most important of these principles is what we call 'The Golden Rule', which is the basis for building the networks of mutual obligation that provide the foundation for community. A sense of mutual obligation can be either specific or general. If it is specific, the reciprocity is specific: I'll do this for you, if you do that for me. If it is general, the reciprocity is generalised. If we do what we can to help other people now, then someday, when we need help, someone may help us. The Golden Rule is a classic call to practice the principle of generalised reciprocity. Moreover, the same call is enunciated, with slight variations, in all of the 11 major religious traditions (Tobias 1995: 124).

In all these traditions, the call for us to practice generalised reciprocity is the same. Table 8.2 presents these 'rules'. There are no short cuts. There are no quick fixes. We cannot hope to develop community in our localities unless we do unto others as *we* would have them do unto *us*.

Politically-committed Dimension of Training

Community development is not only a principle-oriented practice, but is also a political process. It is not a party political process. It is not partisan. It is committed equally to people on both on the left and the right. It is not a state political process. It does not project our problems and the solution of our problems onto the state – quite the contrary. It recognises that if we have problems in our communities then we will have to solve those problems ourselves. However, it is a political process in the sense that it is about empowerment.

Table 8.2   The Golden Rule in the major religions

The Golden Rule	*Hinduism* 'Never do to others what would pain you.' *Panchatantra 3.104*	*Buddhism* 'Hurt not others with that which hurts yourself.' *Udana 5.18*	*Zoroastrianism* 'Do not to others what is not well for oneself.' *Shayast-na-shayast 13.29*
Jainism 'One who neglects existence disregards their own existence.' *Mahavira*	*Confucianism* 'Do not impose on others what you do not yourself desire.' *Analects 12.2*	*Taoism* 'Regard your neighbour's loss or gain as your own loss or gain.' *Tai Shang Kan Ying Pien*	*Baha'i* 'Desire not for any-one the things you would not desire for yourself.' *Baha'Ullah 66*
Judaism 'What is hateful to you do not do to your neighbour.' *Talmud, Shabbat 31a*	*Christianity* 'Do unto others as you would have them do unto you'. *Matthew 7.12*	*Islam* 'Do unto all people as you would they should do to you.' *Mishkat-el-Masabih*	*Sikhism* 'Treat others as you would be treated yourself.' *Adi Granth*

Within my philosophy, I think about two ways of understanding power. Traditionally our notion of power has been defined as the ability to control other people. This tradition emphasises bringing about change through coercion; getting others to change according to our agendas. While the traditional approach advocates taking control of our lives by taking control of others, the alternative approach advocates taking control of our lives by taking control of ourselves. This alternative emphasises bringing change by transformation – encouraging one another to change our lives, individually and collectively, in the light of an agenda of sustainable justice and peace.

The traditional notion of power is popular because it often brings quick, dramatic results. Nevertheless, it is characterised by short-term gains for some, and long-term losses for everyone else. Violent revolutions eventually betray the people in whose names they are fought. The alternative notion of power has been unpopular because it is a slow, unspectacular process. That said, it is slowly but surely gaining in popularity as people begin to realise it is the only way that groups can transcend their selfishness, resolve their conflicts and manage their affairs in a way that achieves justice.

The British community worker, Fred Milson says, our work will be able to be judged to have succeeded or failed, 'by the practical demonstration in all feasible areas, that the community [was able to] define its own needs and organise [its own] resources to satisfy them' (Milson 1974: 26). At the end of the day, our community-based training efforts should be judged in this way.

The Possibility of Transformation through Training

Although it is easy to *teach* about personal integrity and social justice in the classroom, it is difficult, if not impossible, to actually *learn* personal integrity and social justice except in the context of the ebb and flow of ordinary everyday life within community itself. Therefore, we invited students from the colleges where we were teaching to come and live in our community for two or three weeks to *learn* something about personal integrity and social justice.

We introduced them to Aunty Jean, an Aboriginal Elder, who not only told them the story of her people and their painful dispossession but also took them with her to meet her people: some in a maximum security prison, languishing in their cells, and others in a human rights organisation, fighting for their release.

And we introduced them to Father Kefle, an Eritrean priest, who showed them the scars of 30 years of civil war. The students visited refugees who have been torn away from their families, tortured by the very people who were supposed to protect them, forced to flee for their lives, and are now struggling to rebuild a life for themselves as strangers in a strange land.

Some of the students had never actually met an Indigenous Australian or a refugee face-to-face before, let alone heard their story or seen their struggle for themselves. These encounters were confronting for the students who asked the same questions we all need to ask ourselves. How do we, as members of a 'white' society deal with our 'black' history? How do we, as members of the human family respond to the desperate plea from our brothers and sisters, not just to address the superficial symptoms, but the underlying causes, of their ongoing pain? and, What are you – and I – going to do about it? These are questions to us, which call for answers from us; not merely theoretical answers, but practical answers. Answering these questions is a moral imperative that we can accept or reject, but which we cannot ignore.

One of the students who accepted the moral imperative to answer these questions, as honestly as he could, was a police officer who I will call 'Brad', who had been on the police beat for many years. Brad said that he along with many other police officers only related to people in their job as sources of information about 'criminals', or as potential or actual 'criminals', and had become cynical about the public. However, when he took the opportunity to get out of uniform and meet people he had stereotyped face-to-face, as fellow human beings, he began to change. The first stage was 'perspective'. What we see depends on where we stand. For Brad standing with the very people he had often been expected to take a stand against helped him see a different side to the struggle on the streets. The second stage was 'responsibility'. What we hear depends on whom we listen to. When Brad started to listen to people he usually ignored it helped him not only hear a different side to the story of our history, but also to accept his part as a police officer in perpetuating that history. The third stage was 'pain'. How we feel depends on what we do. Recognising that what he was doing as a police officer was often part of the problem, rather than part of the solution, helped Brad feel the impact of the issues much more acutely. The fourth stage was 'responsiveness'. We have two options for managing the pain that comes from recognising the gap between whom we are and who we are meant to be. One option is rationalisation: changing the ideal, so it is closer to whom we are. The other option is transformation: changing the reality, so we are closer to whom we are meant to be.

The chance for Brad to choose transformation rather than rationalisation came along one day when a local Aboriginal person asked him for a smoke. Instead of moving on as he usually did Brad chose to stop and have a smoke and a bit of a chat, like he would have done with any of his other mates. This small change was a big deal for Brad.

This was the stage of 'realisation' Brad was at when he completed the course. I told him how encouraged I was about the stages of change he had gone through, and I encouraged him to take the change a stage further.

The fifth stage of change is 'practice'. We are what we do repeatedly. Transformation is not a single act; rather it is the habitual practice of personal integrity and social justice in our communities. All quality *in situ* community work training provides the opportunity for transformation.

Conclusion

Some sixty years on from starting my journey *in situ* training as a learner, and some forty years on from my journey as an enabler of others' learning, I feel that I have developed a coherent community work training philosophy within my community development work. In reflecting on this philosophy, I am reminded of Parker Palmer (1983), the Quaker community worker saying that education can be driven by either love or fear. Too often training is driven by fear; facilitators in fear of key performance indicators and learners in fear of assessment. For me, at the heart of quality *in situ* community work training situated in the experiential context of the community where the participants live and work together, is the need for the training space to be enchanted with a love that seeks to do justice for one and all.

References

Andrews, D. and Beazley, H. 2010. *Learnings: Lessons We Are Learning About Living Together*. Brisbane: Community Initiatives Resource Centre, Frank Communications.

Clark, D.B. 1975. *Basic Communities: Towards an Alternative Society.* London: Society for Promoting Christian Knowledge.

Covey, S. 1989. *The Seven Habits of Highly Effective People.* New York: Simon and Schuster.

Goleman, D. 1995. *Emotional Intelligence.* New York: Bantam Books.

Macmurray, J. 1968. *Freedom in the Modern World*. London: Faber and Faber.

Milson, F.W. 1974. *An Introduction to Community Work.* London: Routledge and Kegan Paul.

Palmer, P.J. 1983. *To Know As We Are Known: Education as a Spiritual Journey.* San Francisco: Harper and Rowe.

Peck, M.S. 1987. *The Different Drum: Community Making and Peace.* London: Rider and Co.

Putnam, R.D. 2000. *Bowling Alone: The Collapse and Revival of American Community*. New York: Simon & Schuster.

Smith, L.E. 1994. *Intimacy and Mission: Intentional Community as Crucible for Radical Discipleship*. Harrisonburg: Herald Press.

Tobias, M., Morrison, J. and Gray, B. eds 1995. *A Parliament of Souls: In Search of Global Spirituality*. San Francisco: KQED Books.

Vanier, J. 1989. *Community and Growth: Our Pilgramage Together*. New York: Paulist Press.

Vanier, J. 1992. *From Brokenness to Community*. New York: Paulist Press.

Westoby, P., Hope-Simpson, G. and Owen, J. 2009. Stability without strangling: The ongoing story of the Community Initiatives Resource Association, 2003–2008. *New Community Quarterly*, 7(2), 21–5.

PART III
International Stories of Practice

Chapter 9

Strengthening Governance through *Storians:* An Elicitive Approach to Peace-building in Vanuatu

Polly O. Walker

We have bows and we have arrows, and we are skilled in using them. But we can always use a few more arrows.

Chief Selwyn Garu, Malvatumauri National Council of Chiefs

Introduction

The metaphor above captures the elicitive training philosophy, which is the foundation of a series of community-based conflict resolution trainings facilitated through a partnership in Vanuatu. These training workshops, called *storians*, from the Bislama term for 'storying', are central elements of a broader partnership between the Malvatumauri National Council of Chiefs (MNCC), The Australian Centre for Peace and Conflict Studies (ACPACS) at The University of Queensland,[1] and the Australian Government Overseas Aid Program (AusAID). This partnership began in 2005, in response to an invitation from the MNCC for ACPACS' researchers and practitioners to work collaboratively with chiefs to strengthen customary governance, enhancing their capacity to deal with introduced political, social and economic change. Vanuatu has been described as a post-colonial state, dealing with intense and widespread pressures. Ni-Vanuatu[2] also have a long history of dealing creatively to accommodate these changes, building new frameworks and institutions which draw on customary systems and relationships (Westoby 2009). Customary chiefs have been credited for as much as 85 per cent of the security in the region, and their role is enshrined in the Vanuatu Constitution. Nevertheless,

---

1   The Australian Centre for Peace and Conflict Studies (ACPACS) at The University of Queensland operated until 2011 as an autonomous Centre. It has recently been incorporated into The University of Queensland Institute for Social Science Research (ISSR).

2   Ni-Vanuatu is used to refer to all Melanesian ethnicities originating in Vanuatu.

kastom[3] governance, including customary conflict resolution, is struggling to deal with new types of conflicts.

In developing the community-based conflict resolution training, we were aware of the importance of envisioning the process within a broader peace-building framework that would avoid the imposition of Western models of conflict resolution. Over the past 15 years, there have been a growing number of critiques regarding the dominance of Western conflict resolution in international training (Lederach 1995, Kraybill 1996, see Bagshaw 2009, Porter and Bagshaw 2009). In particular, Western conflict resolution models carry a 'residue of imperialism when they attempt to transfer their mediation models to other cultures as the *right* way to resolve conflict [my emphasis]' (Ledearch 1995: 3). The West has the power to maintain these impositions (Galtung 1990: 314), making unreflective conflict resolution training a source of epistemic violence, the marginalisation or suppression of a peoples' way of knowing (Walker 2004).

The field of conflict resolution training is dominated by conflict resolution models arising out of the United States, such as Fisher and Ury's (1981) interest based model, which has been critiqued as smoothing the functioning of the neoliberal systems of governance rather than exposing power imbalances between Western and indigenous systems (Bagshaw 2009). In contrast, conflict resolution training located within a peace-building framework must necessarily build on the strengths of local, traditional practices and give priority to retrieving and reclaiming local epistemologies, customary or 'folk' knowledge about conflict and its resolution (Bagshaw 2009).

Drawing on extant research, we developed the conflict resolution *storians* in ways that challenged hegemonic Western constructs of mediation and mediation training in the Asia-Pacific region by encouraging the use of reflexive approaches, which incorporate the cultural systems of the communities involved, and by working within a framework of social justice and sustainable peace. Members of our partnership believe strongly that *elicitive* approaches, which draw on the knowledge and worldview of participants, address issues both of culture and power, and elide the hegemonic power of Western governance/conflict resolution.

Theoretical Foundations of Cross-cultural Conflict Resolution Training

In developing the *storians* in ways that built respectfully on customary conflict resolution frameworks, we realised that sometimes our understanding might be limited because of worldview differences between and among members of the governance partnership, including *storian* participants. Responding to Michelle LeBaron's (2003) challenge that there are no culturally neutral conflict resolution processes, and that therefore cultural fluency is essential in addressing conflict, we

---

3   *Kastom* is the Bislama term for customary approaches, including *Kastom* law, *Kastom* governance, *Kastom* conflict resolution.

endeavoured to enhance and implement effective worldviewing skills, both within our training teams and in the *storians*.

We were aware that we would be negotiating across worldviews, and that the process was never simple or linear. Not simple, in part because worldviews reside largely as 'the underlying, hidden level of culture' (Hall 1983). Although often out of our conscious awareness, worldviews are powerful, representing the ways cultural groups make sense of the world and decide how to act responsibly and ethically within it – their shared commonsense, so to speak, the deep assumptions that they hold about the world (Avruch and Black 1991: 28).

Worldviews can be also challenging to deal with because most people cannot clearly identify or easily articulate them. Worldviews are lived experience and can often be better understood by watching how people act rather than listening to what they espouse. Worldviews are also challenging to understand because they are constantly changing and being re-negotiated by members of a group. Indeed, a number of worldview scholars explain that it would be more accurate to say that we practice *worldviewing* rather than to say we *have* a worldview. As we interact with others in worldviewing, we collaborate with them to view or make the social worlds in which we live (Docherty 2001: 52).

When many conflict resolution trainers reach the point of understanding that worldviewing involves the out-of-awareness aspects of our experience, and that worldviews are constantly changing, they often place the process in the 'too hard basket' and continue their practice as if their conflict resolution models can 'cut across' cultures with professional techniques. However, ignoring differences in worldview may both cause intercultural conflicts and exacerbate existing conflicts between groups, disrupting or destroying the collaborations that community workers seek to create.

In a worldview conflict, behaviour that is considered appropriate in one worldview is considered disrespectful and disruptive when viewed through the lens of another culture. Our partnership deliberately chose to deal with both the visible and underlying cultural differences in local and Western conflict resolution models. Although we were aware of best practice, and positioned ourselves to deal respectfully and ethically with deep cultural differences, nevertheless we faced a number of worldview conflicts within the partnership. We faced a particularly challenging worldview conflict around finding ways to build mediative capacity in conflicts involving accusations of sorcery, a topic that is seldom addressed or even acknowledged within Western conflict resolution (see Walker and Garu 2009).

In building effective worldviewing skills, with the intent of voicing the out-of-awareness aspects of Ni-Vanuatu conflict resolution, we chose to base our training primarily on an elicitive training model. Our elicitive training model considered as foundational the rich resource of *kastom* conflict resolution in Vanuatu, which represents a wide range of peacemaking processes taking place both in urban and rural settings. The *storians* have been designed to elicit fuller descriptions, understandings and articulations of *kastom* mediation, to introduce frameworks of Western mediation, to explore particular skills and processes within Western mediation and to analyse the ways that introduced institutions have impacted on *kastom* mediation. The *storians* also facilitate the exploration of ways in which the integration of Western skills and processes might enhance the mediative capacity of Ni-Vanuatu chiefs and community leaders.

In collaboratively developing the *storians* with the MNCC, we conceptualised our approach as building stronger *mediative capacity*, 'helping particular institutions within the wider society to build ... attitudes, skills, and disciplines that include engagement of the diverse perspectives about a conflict' (Lederach 2005: 95–6). Although there are a number of conflict resolution scholars (see Lederach 1995, Porter and Bagshaw 2009) who argue for the importance of *elicitive* processes which draw on local indigenous conflict knowledge and practice, the majority of international conflict resolution training is *prescriptive* – built on the premise of transferring knowledge from expert trainer to local consumers. In *prescriptive* training, the expertise of the trainers shapes the framework and process of training and local indigenous knowledge is subsumed into the trainers' explicit, 'expert' knowledge. The main purpose of prescriptive training is to share a practice framework and train participants in how to implement the model.

In contrast, an *elicitive* training approach considers training to be an opportunity to discover, create, and solidify conflict resolution models which emerge from the cultural resources of the participants and which respond to local needs in particular contexts (Lederach 1995: 55). The ACPACS team felt strongly that, given the brief to strengthen local and customary conflict resolution capacity, an elicitive training approach was necessary. The role of trainers was seen as catalysts and facilitators, not as experts. This allowed the participants to articulate their own ethnoconflict theory, their conceptualisations of what constitutes conflict and how it might be processed in ways that support their own values and beliefs (Avruch and Black 1991).

Previously in this chapter, I described the epistemic violence of imposing Western prescriptive style training in the Pacific Islands. Regardless of the limitations of a prescriptive approach, quite often the most beneficial training incorporates a blend of both elicitive and prescriptive processes, with the balance designed to address the needs of the community (Lederach 1995).

Continuing to explore the theoretical foundation of community-based cross-cultural conflict resolution training, I will now discuss the five steps in Lederach's elicitive conflict resolution training (1995: 58–61) model. To help illustrate these steps I will also describe some of the activities we facilitated as part of each step in a conflict resolution *storian* in Port Vila. Woven into the five steps are three guiding principles (Lederach 1995: 110–15):

- *Conflict* 'in situ': the need for inquisitiveness about what currently exists in a community.
- *Indigenous empowerment*: people in the setting are considered to be the key resources in the training.
- *Conscientisation:* awareness of self-in-context, based on the belief that people are capable of understanding and naming the conflicts they face

and their conflict resolution processes. This is a paradoxical approach, which 'invites a particular group to reflect within itself on the strengths and weaknesses of its own heritage, knowledge, and modalities related to conflict' (Lederach 1995: 113).

The five steps which support these three principles are as follows:

Step One: Discovery

This is aimed at facilitating participants' engagement with their own conflict knowledge and increasing respect for their knowledge as a valuable resource. On day one of the *storian*, after an opening ceremony, we explored the reasons why we were there, explaining that we respected participants' knowledge of conflict resolution and would be working with them on strengthening customary and local processes. We elicited participants' knowledge about the interconnections between conflict and governance, exploring different levels of Ni-Vanuatu governance (local, island, province, state). Participants were asked to explore/ assess the forces of change that were disrupting the order and organisation of their communities, and the conflicts that were arising out of those disruptions. When reporting back, participants described the strength of customary conflict resolution and explored its weaknesses in dealing with some conflicts involving international actors/institutions, introduced frameworks and institutions, and women and youth. Participants also expressed a desire to learn new skills which would enhance their conflict resolution processes in these situations.

Step Two: Naming

Participants are encouraged to define and name their own processes/frameworks. *Storian* participants formed groups based on their province. They were asked to share their metaphors for conflict, and for conflict resolution, building on the principle that out-of-awareness aspects of worldview are more easily and quickly reached through metaphor, narrative and other aesthetic forms than through linear analysis. After some discussion about, and playing around with, the meaning of *metaphor*, some of the chiefs said, 'Ah, in Bislama, this would be *tok picture*' or a picture that talks, sharing a deeper story or meaning. After participants drew detailed and intricate metaphors of conflict resolution, it became clear that, although there were underlying commonalities in worldview, the different provinces had different processes of dealing with conflict. At the end of this session, the *nakamal*[4] was filled with elaborate drawings hanging on the wall and the murmur of voices as people appreciatively examined their own, and others' pictorial representations of conflict resolution.

---

4   In this context *Nakamal* refers to a gathering place.

Next, we invited participants to explore and answer the following questions, with the intent of beginning to articulate models of conflict resolution for each of the provinces:

- Entry into conflict resolution: Who will be involved? Where? How will we manage the process?
- How do we find out what happened to create the conflict?
- How do learn more about where are we in the conflict?
- How do we get out of the conflict? How do we transform it?
- Resolution/transformation: What does it look like? How is it recorded/ disseminated? Who is responsible for what actions in implementing the resolution? (Lederach 1995).

After each of these activities (drawing metaphors and articulating the five aspects of a conflict resolution framework) we briefly compared and contrasted Western metaphors for conflict resolution and Western frameworks of conflict resolution, discussing their strengths and limitations among the wider Australian community, and in other countries.

Step Three – Evaluation

Participants were encouraged to evaluate the effectiveness of *kastom* conflict resolution in particular contexts, and describe points at which it was ineffective. They also discussed strategies, which might be implemented when *kastom* processes are not equipped to address contemporary conflicts.

Facilitators explained that the *storian* was designed in part to share new conflict resolution skills which might be used to address conflicts which customary approaches were not designed to deal with. Moreover, the new skills were not to replace or suppress *kastom*, but rather to build on its strong foundation. At this point, Chief Selwyn Garu shared with participants his metaphor of 'a few more arrows' (which opens this chapter), explaining how new skills could enhance customary conflict resolution.

At the end of the day, ACPACS facilitators met with Ni-Vanuatu facilitators, who had led all of the small group sessions. We gathered to hear feedback, share experiences and plan for the next day. On the first day of this *storian*, Ni-Vanuatu facilitators primarily described the participants' enthusiastic participation. However, they reported that a small group of high-ranking chiefs were very upset about the process. In the final section of this chapter, I will explore the conflict which arose and how we addressed it.

At the beginning of day two, we introduced Johan Galtung's peace-building grid (as shown in Table 9.1) which provided a format through which participants could explore both positive and negative aspects of conflict resolution as it has occurred in Ni-Vanuatu governance in the past, and how it might be envisioned for the future. Participants used this grid to evaluate some of the types of conflicts

Table 9.1   Galtung's peace-building grid

	Negative	Positive
Future	(4) Potential or actual problems, difficulties	(1) Vision/Options Desirable possibilities
Past/ Present	(2) Traumatic Memory(ies), Experiences	(3) Past Pleasures-satisfactions

taking place in their communities. They worked with practice stories involving mediation within the *nakamal* and conflict resolution in the local community. Through this exploration, they developed a written expression of Ni-Vanuatu conflict management frameworks, including the stages or steps they would go through in managing conflict within their preferred futures, and in relation to different levels of governance. Participants then compared and contrasted their current conflict resolution processes with their preferred future vision.

Step Four – Adapt/Recreate

These are processes of adapting existing conflict resolution models to meet contemporary conflicts. We introduced a tool for analysing conflict to explore: which parties were involved in the conflict; what positions they had taken in relation to the conflict; what emotions they were experiencing around the conflict; and what their needs and underlying values were in relation to the conflict.

On days three and four of the training, we worked primarily in adapting and recreating local Ni-Vanuatu conflict resolution models. We demonstrated and discussed skills drawn from Western conflict resolution, including: deep listening, summarising so that people know they were heard, identifying positions/ interests/ values and dealing with difficult people. Participants engaged in role play, games and outdoor activities to explore how these and other conflict resolution skills might assist in dealing with community conflicts. Participants also critiqued Western conflict resolution in terms of what would work in Vanuatu. While there was agreement that the entire model would not work it was felt that some of the skills used within it had potential for empowering Ni-Vanuatu to deal more effectively with contemporary and introduced conflicts.

Step Five – Practical Application

This involves experimenting with and refining emerging models. On the final day of the *storian*, participants worked in their groups to create action plans for strengthening conflict resolution in communities in their provinces. Drawing on the elicited frameworks and models of conflict resolution, each group developed a plan that specified who would be involved in resolving conflict, what they would do, when the process would take place, and how it would be evaluated to develop sustainable conflict resolution.

While the five steps and the examples presented here suggest an easy and logical flow, the work of community-based cross-cultural conflict resolution training is rarely so straightforward. In the next section of this chapter, I share two practice stories drawn from our collaborative partnership, which illustrate both the strengths and challenges of training processes embedded in local knowledge and culture.

Practice Stories: Evaluating Elicitive Style Training within the Vanuatu Partnership

Although we felt confident that we had drawn on the most rigorous extant research, we were at times surprised at the outcomes of the *storians*. We were challenged to implement 'navigational capacity' (Arai 2006: 76–79), 'our awareness of both the challenges and opportunities presented' in a cross-cultural training context, including how we could respond in ways that created interdependence. This section focuses on two practice stories which explore the nexus of elicitive training and cross cultural communication. The first example illustrates strengths of the training process – how the skills being taught in one of the *storians* were immediately integrated to successfully and creatively transform a conflict among participants in the *storian*. The second story demonstrates the entanglement between elicitive training and effective cross-cultural communication, including the challenges posed in navigating across different worldviews.

Practice Story One

At the closing ceremony of the 2007 *storian* in Port Vila, Chief Selwyn brought one of the women leaders up to the ACPACS facilitators, saying 'This woman has something important to tell you.' She was a member of a group that met each day under the Nambanga tree in the front of the *nakamal*. Earlier that day, their group had stayed outside under the tree while the other groups came into the *nakamal* for the final session. We needed all groups to finalise their action plans for the conflict resolution projects they were designing. As I started to speak with them, they suddenly broke into a loud, repetitive chant that echoed across the grounds and through the *nakamal*. At the time, we all wondered what was going on. Now the participant smiled and explained what had happened, saying:

> We are all members of a political party and we are from different sides of a
> split that has divided the party in two. Now we found ourselves at this *storian*,
> and we were learning new mediation skills so we thought, why not put them
> into practice? We decided that we would all meet together at lunch, under the
> Nambanga tree, and we would practice what we had learned during the day and
> see if it could help resolve the conflict between us. On Tuesday, we used the

conflict web to analyse the interests and needs of all the parties in our conflict. On Wednesday, we sat and we practiced listening for the roots of the problem, for the underlying issues. It went okay. On Thursday, we continued, and things got pretty heated. One of the chiefs stood up and was so angry he wanted to hit another guy, but we practiced what we had explored about dealing with difficult people, and in a bit, the angry chief calmed down, and we continued to talk. Today at lunch, we reconciled. That is what you heard when you came out to greet us. We were singing the chant of our political party to show that we are united once again.

This story illustrates participants' particularly powerful and effective integration of new skills into existing relationships and processes, resulting in the transformation of an entrenched conflict. We would not necessarily expect such a rapid change to take place, particularly in a training setting, and probably would advise against implementing skills without careful reflection. Nevertheless, local actors, building on their knowledge of relationships, 'right time', process and setting were able to peacefully transform a conflict.

Not all of our training experiences were immediately successful. We also experienced challenges which threatened to create new conflicts, as will become evident in the second practice story.

Practice Story Two

In 2007, our partnership began to provide training for Ni-Vanuatu facilitators, with the intent of Ni-Vanuatu taking over the facilitation of *storians* after a period of co-training with ACPACS facilitators. We first held a five-day conflict resolution train-the-trainer *storian*, in this case a double storied process of exploring Ni-Vanuatu conflict transformation while at the same time training Ni-Vanuatu in culturally appropriate principles and processes of adult learning. The week went well, with Ni-Vanuatu facilitators eagerly exploring ways in which participants could draw on their own culture, knowledge, wisdom and practice. The participants were also encouraged to explore and critique new skills and processes, with the intent of developing a syncretic form of conflict resolution, one based in customary cultural values and ways of knowing, yet responsive to conflicts induced in part by introduced systems. On Monday of the second week, we were set for a large conflict transformation *storian* including forty or more chiefs and community leaders. Our process was, after introduction by Malvatumauri Council of Chiefs, for the three ACPACS facilitators to take a lead in large group facilitation, and Ni-Vanuatu facilitators to take over facilitation of activities/processes with small groups of participants. The first day, drawing on what we considered to be the most rigorous research in conflict transformation training, we worked primarily in an elicitive mode. We asked participant groups to create and draw metaphors for resolving conflict. They also created lists of values that underlie customary peacemaking. The day went on in this manner, with a growing number of sheets of butcher's paper adorning the walls of the *nakamal* as groups finished their work and put it up for the other groups to view while they discussed it. At the day's end, the ACPACS facilitators met with the Ni-Vanuatu facilitators to debrief the day, to find out what went well, what could be improved, and importantly, what happened in the small groups facilitated by Ni-Vanuatu trainers. The Ni-Vanuatu facilitators were enthused about the day, the knowledge that had been elicited, and the unfolding process designed to lead to the creation of action plans for strengthening Ni-Vanuatu conflict resolution processes. The Ni-Vanuatu facilitators cautioned us, however, that a small number of higher ranking chiefs had challenged them, saying that they believed the Malvatumauri had brought Australian facilitators to Port Vila to 'steal their knowledge.' This group of chiefs pointed out that a great deal of their *kastom* knowledge regarding conflict and peacemaking was posted up on the walls for all to see. They also argued that the Australian facilitators had shared very little new information, and it appeared that they had come, as had so many people before, to steal what was of great value to the chiefs and Ni-Vanuatu people and to take it overseas.

We were crestfallen and dismayed; our intentions, based on what we considered to be the best research and practice paradigms, had backfired with these participants, having the exact opposite outcome of what was desired in regard to respect for indigenous knowledge. The Ni-Vanuatu facilitators said however, 'We told the chiefs that you were not stealing knowledge. We explained that we had just completed a week of training that covered the same material they would be covering, and that if they just came back and gave it a chance, they would see that the purpose was to strengthen Ni-Vanuatu peacemaking.'

We discussed what might be done to shift this situation, and decided that the next morning we would move quickly into exploring Western conflict resolution skills and processes, and build a foundation for critical analysis of culturally appropriate conflict resolution.

The next morning, we once again briefly described elicitive training, explaining that we were not claiming to be experts in the best conflict resolution process for Ni-Vanuatu. We emphasised that participants held the most valuable knowledge about conflict resolution in their context, but that we were experienced in research and practice of Western conflict resolution and would share knowledge regarding these processes. We explained that the new skills we were sharing were intended for participant groups to practice, critique and evaluate in relation to their appropriateness in the Ni-Vanuatu context. In addition, we explained that the *kastom* knowledge elicited in the group activities would stay with the group, and that the drawings, lists and other visuals posted on the walls would stay within Vanuatu and would not be taken to Australia. We then proceeded into a number of interactive processes throughout the day which explored skills drawn from Western conflict resolution.

At the end of the second day, the Ni-Vanuatu facilitators said that everything was fine, that all of the participants were satisfied with how the *storian* was progressing, including the chiefs who had expressed concerns. We went on with a very intense week of facilitation as we negotiated across worldviews. On the afternoon of the final day we arrived at the time for the closing ceremony.

The closing ceremonies of the *storians* are always rich with ritual, ceremony, laughter, appreciation, and performance, followed by a great feast. Everyone, including the facilitators, looks forward to them with great anticipation. On this day, we were all assembled in the *nakamal*, ready to begin the celebrations, when one of the chiefs (from the previously concerned group) stood up and said, 'Wait. We cannot begin this ceremony which will signify we have all completed this *storian* and will now commit ourselves to peacemaking. We cannot create peace in Vanuatu if we do not have peace in this *nakamal*. We accused the Malvatumauri of something that was not true, and we must make it right, so that we are reconciled here, in this gathering.'

The four chiefs who had earlier expressed concerns about our 'stealing knowledge' came forward with finely woven mats and asked Chief Selwyn to come forward. They placed the mats on the floor, and Chief Selwyn circled them several times, head bowed, and arms behind his back. The previously aggrieved chiefs then said, 'It is finished; we are reconciled. Now we can begin the closing ceremony in peace. We can now say with truth that we are peacemakers.'

Although this worldview conflict was resolved by the end of the *storian*, it demonstrates the delicate balance involved in negotiating different traditions of knowledge management when engaging in cross-cultural training. On one hand, contemporary research on conflict resolution training in the Asia-Pacific region strongly maintains that *elicitive* style training is essential if conflict resolution is to foster social justice and peace-building. However, in this scenario, our facilitation of *elicitive* processes actually caused a conflict (or brought a latent conflict to the surface). My analysis is that the conflict was in part based in the historical and contemporary disregard of many Western researchers, practitioners and entrepreneurs who have come, and continue to come, to Vanuatu to work and benefit from natural, social and cultural riches, yet give little in return. This has been the case so often that no outside entities are allowed to do research in Vanuatu without the express consent of the Vanuatu Cultural Centre. Our partnership was well aware of these power dynamics, and endeavoured to deal with them. However, positioning ourselves in this way did not remove us from the broader network of power relationships within Vanuatu. As ACPACS facilitators, we could see how the concerned chiefs might have arrived at the conclusion that once again, people had come from outside to benefit from Ni-Vanuatu knowledge. We redoubled our efforts at more clearly articulating our approach to *elicitive* training, and explaining why the partnership thought this was an effective process for the *storians*. To demonstrate our commitment to sharing new skills we moved immediately into a prolonged series of activities which shared, explored and critiqued new knowledge and new conflict resolution skills. In other words, we endeavoured to strengthen our expressive capacity regarding our own cultural perspectives, a critical skill in cultural fluency (Arai 2006).

In some respects, this scenario depicts a worldview conflict around what constituted ethical behaviour as it relates to customary knowledge. Although members of the partnership were clear in their intent to deal respectfully with customary knowledge, participants' had many experiences with members of Western worldviews in which 'expert' knowledge subsumed local knowledge as raw data rather than engaging dialogically with it as equal knowledge systems. In contrast to many Western trainers, ACPACS facilitators took a stance of engaging respectfully with customary knowledge as holding the expertise for effective contemporary conflict resolution. However, on day one of the *storian*, before stronger relationships could be built, and worldviews negotiated, it is reasonable that participants could assume that all Western facilitators subscribed to this aspect of Western worldview. We were challenged to practice ethical worldviewing, to realise that '...that the people of this planet don't just live in one world but in many worlds and some of these worlds, if not properly understood, can and do annihilate the others' (Hall 1983: 200–201).

Conclusion

International conflict resolution training has been justifiably criticised for its reliance on prescriptive processes which marginalise the role of local knowledge and skill in transforming conflict. In contrast, conflict resolution training within a peace-building framework requires respectful engagement with community and customary processes and with frameworks of dealing with conflict. The *Kastom* Governance Partnership has elected to implement community-based elicitive training, which builds on local frameworks of managing conflict. This is achieved by drawing on strengths of customary conflict resolution, naming local processes, reflecting on their limitations in addressing contemporary conflicts, adapting customary models by integrating new skills, and experimenting with the refined models.

Members of the *Kastom* Governance Partnership have demonstrated largely successful negotiation of worldviews, of communicating across differences in underlying aspects of culture, to facilitate effective training. However, these elicitive style trainings have not been without their own challenges, as members of the partnership grapple with a historical context of marginalisation and suppression of customary knowledge, as well as with the integration of conflict resolution issues that seem taboo in Western conflict resolution.

Collaborative, elicitive style training processes have demonstrated capacity to reduce structural violence toward local and indigenous knowledge, to create interdependent and respectful relationships, and to navigate the turbulent waters of cross-cultural communication and conflict resolution.

References

Arai, T. 2006. A journey toward cultural fluency , in *Conflict Across Cultures: A Unique Experience of Bridging Differences*, edited by M. LeBaron and V. Pillay. Boston: Intercultural Press, 57–82.

Avruch, K. and Black, P. 1991. The culture question and conflict resolution. *Peace & Change*, 16(1), 22–45.

Bagshaw, D. 2009. Challenging Western Constructs of Mediation , in *Mediation in the Asia-Pacific Region*, edited by D. Bagshaw and E. Porter. New York: Routledge, 13–30.

Docherty, J.S. 2001. *Learning Lessons from Waco: When the Parties Bring their Gods to the Negotiation Table*. Syracuse: Syracuse University Press.

Fisher, R. and Ury, W. 1981. *Getting to Yes: Negotiating Agreement Without Giving In*. Boston: Penguin.

Galtung, J. 1990. International development in human perspective , in *Conflict: Human Needs Theory*, edited by J.W. Burton. London: Macmillan Press, 301–35.

Galtung, J. 1996. *Peace by Peaceful Means: Peace and Conflict, Development, and Civilization*. Oslo: International Peace Research Institute.

Hall, E.T. 1983. *The Dance of Life*. New York: Anchor Books.

Kraybill, R. 1996. Elicitive training: Dealing with conflict cross-culturally. *Conflict Resolution News*, June, 22–3.

LeBaron, M. 2003. *Bridging Cultural Conflicts: A New Approach for a Changing World* San Francisco: Jossey-Bass.

Lederach, J.P. 1995. *Preparing for Peace: Conflict Transformation Across Cultures*. Syracuse: Syracuse University Press.

Lederach, J.P. 2005. *The Moral Imagination: The Art and Soul of Building Peace*. Oxford: Oxford University Press.

Porter E. and Bagshaw, D. 2009. Transforming conflicts and building peace through mediation , in *Mediation in the Asia-Pacific Region*, edited by D. Bagshaw and E. Porter. New York: Routledge, 6–10.

Walker, P. 2004. Decolonizing conflict resolution: Addressing the ontological violence of Westernization, *American Indian Quarterly*, 28(3–4), 527–49.

Walker, P. and Garu, S. 2009. A few more arrows: Strengthening meditative capacity in Vanuatu, in *Mediation in the Asia-Pacific Region*, edited by D. Bagshaw and E. Porter. New York: Routledge, 94–110.

Westoby, P. 2010. Community-based training for conflict prevention in Vanuatu: Reflections of a practitioner-researcher. *Social Alternatives*, 29(1), 15–19.

Chapter 10

Creativity and Technique: A Participatory Approach to Farmer Education in Cambodia

Nicholas Haines[1]

Introduction

A slightly scruffy-looking man, maybe thirty-seven to thirty-eight years old, stands before the group. He sports the kind of light beard that, whenever *I* grow one, earns me gentle rebukes of *min se-aart* [not beautiful] from my many Cambodian aunts and sisters at the market. He is about to present a poem that his small group laboured over for almost an hour. They huddled over a notebook first, scribbling thoughts and striking things out, talking and testing and taming their words, until finally, the thinking done and the decisions made, they wrote their creation on a flipchart. Even this last step took longer than usual, the humble marker pen wielded as a calligrapher's brush, the poem rendered stroke by stroke, letter by letter, line by line, with exquisite symmetry and care.

The man reads gingerly, as though the words are not his own, as though the words are his master. After the first line, he suddenly stops reading and starts singing, his tone rising and falling lyrically in each line, his volume changing slightly at times to shape a phrase, his vocal chords adding a trill or a flourish here and there. The words emerge on *his* command; they march to a rhythm of *his* making – a rhythm that spreads through the audience as bodies start to rock and eyes start to close. The lines cohere through rhymes that loop back and forth, tying the thoughts together.

The poem conjures an image of what the future could hold – of what an ideal relationship between the people of this village and their closest level of local government, the commune council, would look like. The people would talk with each other about the problems they face as a community; they would make the time to do this even though everyone is busy growing crops and running businesses and raising families. They would agree on a problem that ranks higher than the others do in importance for the village. They would decide what action the commune council should take to respond to this problem. They would present a shared position with compelling reasons to the commune council. The commune councillors, for their part, would invite the people to meetings to discuss the people's concerns and the council's development budget and plans. They would never rest in their efforts to serve the people. They would help the people with

---

1   Nicholas can be emailed at: nicholas.haines@uqconnect.edu.au

every difficulty. They would honour their leadership roles. The people would respond to this behaviour with respect and gratitude, and with wishes for the everlasting happiness of their leaders.

The whole group – about twenty farmers in all, mostly female – buzzes with conversation. My Khmer colleague, the main facilitator of this workshop, poses reflection questions: What meaning did you take from the poem? How did you feel while listening to it? What do the people do in the poem? What do the commune councillors do? What do the people think and feel about the commune councillors, and vice versa? What similarities do you see in the visions of all three small groups who presented today: the group who composed and recited a poem, the group who prepared and performed a short play, the group who drew and explained a picture? My colleague's questions structure a conversation that is already alive. The words tumble out, comments provoke more comments. The geometry of the conversation moves: a one-on-one exchange while everyone else listens; another person joins to form a trio; an idea resonates and almost all speak; two people break off from the group and have a quiet side conversation.

My colleague closes the session with an apt summary and a deft link to the first session: a mini-lecture and an active quiz about Cambodia's decentralisation reforms. He describes the reforms as a chance for people and commune councillors to recast their relationship – to nudge it just a little bit closer to the future we all imagined in our visioning exercise today.

The farmer whose home we are using as a workshop venue is a leader in his community and a farmer trainer in our project. He stands, beams, and takes a photo of the poem with his mobile phone.

The Context

My three Khmer colleagues are a project team in a small Cambodian non-government organisation (NGO) called Srer Khmer. The project trains farmers in agricultural techniques and helps farmers to form farmer associations – a type of legally recognised community-based organisation in which members save money, take out low interest loans and discuss shared concerns. My colleagues work with 20 farmer associations in 20 villages in Banteay Meanchey Province, northwest Cambodia. In 2011, the donor asked Srer Khmer to add another activity to the project: a one-day workshop for each of the 20 farmer associations to raise awareness of Cambodia's decentralisation reforms.

I am a community development advisor to my colleagues. My accordion-like portfolio expands and contracts in response to Srer Khmer's needs, but recently my job has been to craft learning processes through which my colleagues gain not only a wider repertoire of training methods, but a larger imagination of what training can be.

Imaginative training is difficult to do in Cambodia, where learning is generally understood as a process of copying from authority figures. In this context, to train is to lecture – to speak the material for learners to copy. Brainstorming and question and answer activities are sometimes included in the name of participation, but these are used to expedite the copying process, not to foster independent questioning and critical thinking. The trainer is wholly responsible for the learning process. The trainer sees the participants as lacking capacity, particularly if the participants are poor and have low levels of formal education. An instinct to instruct pervades the trainer's practice. The participants are passive and sit in rows like children in a classroom. They accept their capacity-deprived status and defer uncritically to the trainer's expertise.

These ideas about the roles of trainers and participants show up in the strong element of ceremony to most training events in Cambodia. The event is valued more as a symbol of learning than as a space for real learning. Participants regard training events as rituals to observe out of respect for the authority figures who invited them, or out of gratitude to an organisation that has helped them in the past. The measure of a good training event is whether everyone performed their culturally assigned role in the social hierarchy. Did the trainers establish their authority by imparting a body of principles and terminology? Did the trainers keep the participants occupied for the duration of the training? Did the participants turn up and follow instructions? When asked what they learned from the training, participants usually list the names of the sessions – 'I learned about training needs analysis' – rather than name something specific that was important to them personally. This is usually because the training did not trigger new insights, change perceptions or build skills. Another reason is that even if learning did take place, participants struggle to name their learning themselves. They are used to a teacher or trainer doing this for them.

This chapter is about how my colleagues and I wrestled with this context: a context so unfavourable for the kinds of community-based training explored in this book that at times I had no choice but to leave training practice aside and be content with other parts of my job. It tells how we swept aside the obstacles in our path and prised open a space for different concepts of training. It tells a story of struggle and learning and hope.

I begin this chapter with a reflection on how the participatory techniques from my opening story used creativity to connect the participants to each other and to the content of the training, blazing a trail towards a deeper, more meaningful participation. I follow this with a reflection on how my colleagues, through the process of learning participatory techniques, cultivated the art of questioning and improved their training practice. This leads into a discussion of participatory learning and action (PLA): a conceptual framework that helps me make sense of the process my colleagues and I went through. I conclude with a reflection on how I deal with the limitations of participatory learning and action as a training framework.

From Shallow Discussion to Deep Creativity: Remaking Participation

Participatory techniques, particularly those with a creative element, change the pattern of participation by captivating and connecting with people in ways that abstract discussions and dot points cannot. The poetry group from my opening story were enthusiastic about their task; this is obvious from their plea to the facilitator for more time to complete it. I have observed many workshops that assigned a question to a small group and had them discuss it and summarise their thoughts as dot points on a flipchart. That task does not summon the depth of commitment the poetry group showed. Had we used the conventional method the group would have been eager to finish as quickly as possible. The thoroughness of the group's process – the drafting and re-drafting, the lively conversation – and the pride with which they wrote the final version of their work tells me that the task excited the group. It excited them because it was both novel and familiar at the same time. It was novel because they had never done this in a workshop before. It was familiar because it appealed to their experience of folk poetry and other oral traditions.

The process of composing the poem bonded the group members in a shared task that was fun and made sense to them. It made it easier for them to engage with the content of the exercise. Their vision of a good relationship between the people and the commune council leapt from their imaginations onto the page, before soaring to lyrical heights when the man sang it. A conventional discussion culminating in a dot point summary would have obscured that vision, not brought it into focus. Such an exercise would have been too bland and abstract. The medium of poetry, with its lyricism and vivid images, infused the vision with clarity.

The man who sang the poem saw the potential of poetry to liberate him from reading, a task that constrains him. The exercise gave him the chance to move out of the domain of the development worker (reading from a flipchart) and into terrain that is more meaningful to his own experience (singing a folk poem). He seized that chance instinctively. He did not need an invitation. Such is the power of participatory techniques to connect with people on *their* terms.

The poem evoked a deep response from the listeners. People in the audience rocked their bodies gently to the poem's rhythm. They closed their eyes to savour the pleasing sounds and the rich images. It was a stark contrast with audience reactions when a small group reports a dot point list to the whole group. In those situations it is common for listeners to zone out. Some yawn openly, others stare blankly, their minds on the threshold between wakefulness and sleep. I have seen people chain-smoke so that at least their hands are active even if their brains are not. That did not happen in this workshop.

The whole group discussion pulsed with energy because of the emotional experience everyone had shared in listening to the poem. To be moved by a thing of beauty is to acknowledge a part of yourself you cannot control. It is to discard pretence, let down your guard, and be authentic. When the participants saw each other in that state the level of safety in the group rose, emboldening the quieter people to participate in the discussion. Through that shared experience of authenticity the participants gave themselves and each other permission to speak up. Most of the group discussions I have seen in Cambodia are not true group discussions: almost all of the interaction is between the facilitator and a handful of confident participants. This workshop was different.

The farmer trainer's act of photographing the poem grabbed my attention. The poem so moved him – and he was so proud of the work of his peers – that he wanted to capture it for posterity. Other workshops produce thick sheaves of flipchart paper that gather dust in desk drawers. This workshop produced something worth preserving.

The effect of the techniques on the participants was obvious. The effect on my colleagues' training practice was more subtle, but no less important.

From Testing Recall to Honouring Stories: Cultivating the Art of Questioning

The process of learning the participatory techniques of a visioning exercise changed my Khmer colleagues' training practice more deeply than I expected. In the workshop description that opened this chapter, my colleague posed reflective questions that sound unremarkable. These are standard questions to ask if you are a participatory trainer. Yet those questions reveal a profound change in the way my colleague trains.

When I started working with my Khmer colleagues, they would ask questions to test farmers' ability to recall a concept or recite a term my colleagues had presented rather than to elicit thoughts, evoke feelings or invite analysis. I first realised that this was their understanding of what questions are for when I joined them on field trips for a baseline study about a year before the workshop. One of the questions in our questionnaire survey was: *In your opinion, who is the real owner of the farmer association in your village? Why do you feel this way?* I had included this question in the survey because I wanted to find out how the farmers saw their stake in their farmer association (FA). In the first few villages everyone gave the standard response, 'We all own the FA because we discuss everything together'. This is what the FAs are supposed to be like. The reality is usually different, with the FAs depending heavily on the authority of Srer Khmer staff, or the charisma and energy of a FA office-bearer, to get things done. The FA office-bearers – the chairman, the secretary, and the treasurer – would often ask my colleagues to set dates for FA meetings because otherwise the FA members would not turn up. FA members would sometimes ask my colleagues to resolve their crisis of confidence in their office-bearers, or to take charge of their FA's finances because they no longer trusted their treasurer.

One day a respondent answered the question differently. She said Srer Khmer is the real owner of the FA in her village. I was intrigued, and looked forward to hearing her reasons for seeing it that way. But my colleague did not ask the follow-up question about the respondent's reasons. Instead, she responded with a lecture about how FAs belong to the members. The respondent agreed meekly and my colleague duly recorded the revised response. I asked my colleague to pause, pointing out that a minute ago the respondent named Srer Khmer as the real owner of the FA. 'She changed her mind', was my colleague's reply. I countered, 'She changed her mind based on what you said. We cannot change the data we don't like. That isn't research.' My colleague asked the follow-up question about the respondent's original answer. The respondent explained that she regards Srer Khmer as the real owner of the FA because Srer Khmer formed the FA and provides advice and training to it.

Over lunch, I chatted with another colleague who had been conducting interviews by himself in the same village that morning. I asked about responses to the question about FA ownership and was told, 'Oh, they were confused. They think Srer Khmer is the real owner. I told them they were wrong.'

I despaired about the quality of our data. However, I decided to use the incident as a learning moment. I explained that there are no right or wrong answers to a question about a person's opinions or interpretations. We want to know what the respondents really think so that we can improve our work. The study will be useless as a learning tool if we change the data to fit what we want to hear.

Over the next few weeks my colleagues contained their urge to correct responses, and they explored the respondents' thinking. They heard proof that farmers' thoughts and experiences are diverse and worth asking about. Their concept of knowledge changed. They moved from assuming knowledge to be universally true and external to the knower to entertaining the thought that some forms of knowledge depend on context and are created by the knower. However, I sensed that although they *apprehended* the point, they did not *comprehend* it. Their response was, 'Yes, I see what you're saying. I take your point.' But the point did not fit into their mental maps for organising their development practice. They had not made this new learning their own. Their motive for changing their interviewing technique was to comply with someone else's vision – my vision – of good research practice. I had imposed knowledge on them before they perceived the need for it. My intentions were good: I wanted our research to be rigorous and useful. And I succeeded in raising the standard of our study. But I had not crafted a learning process through which my colleagues could discover their need for new knowledge. Inadvertently, I had repeated the very teaching pattern I was trying to transform!

That changed when I introduced my colleagues to the participatory techniques of a visioning exercise. In our first six workshops about Cambodia's decentralisation reforms we did not have a visioning exercise. We followed the lecture about decentralisation with small group discussions about the benefits people can get from participating in commune planning. This merely led to lists of infrastructure: roads, canals, farm ponds, schools, health centres. It did not advance people's thinking or uncover new insights. After the first six workshops we had a two-week break from training. We spent some of that time reflecting on how the workshops were going and analysing the strengths and weaknesses of our workshop design. Our workshop included a problem tree exercise for analysing constraints to popular participation in commune planning. The recurring theme from this exercise the first six times was the poor quality of the relationship between citizens and their commune councils. The parties to the relationship do not understand each other, do not trust each other, do not empathise with each other's needs and situations. My colleagues decided to make this theme the central problem in the problem tree exercise in the remaining 14 workshops. Participants would analyse the causes of the current, deeply flawed relationship; this would lead into an action planning exercise in which participants agreed on realistic first steps they could take to address a key issue from the analysis.

That is when I saw the relevance of a visioning exercise before the problem tree exercise. The visioning exercise could invite people to imagine what an ideal relationship between citizens and commune councils would look like. This would build a shared agenda for the workshop: a common goal for everyone to work toward. It would be more useful than compiling shopping lists of infrastructure.

I shared my thought with my colleagues and gained their permission for us to practise what I was talking about. Two of my colleagues drew a picture that showed their vision of an ideal relationship between the people and the commune council. My other colleague and I prepared and performed a short play for the same purpose.

After doing the exercise we practised asking reflection questions. At that point, posing those questions was not merely something I was urging my colleagues to do. The questions emerged naturally from the exercise. Questions about what happened, and what people noticed and how people acted make sense after an exercise built around a living story. If there are real people doing real things, there is something tangible to unpack through reflection questions. Questions about feelings are relevant after an exercise that evoked feelings. Through learning the techniques of a visioning exercise, my colleagues realised their need for the skill of posing reflection questions. This made it possible for them to fit this new knowledge into the conceptual frameworks they already held.

The techniques were my colleagues' entry point to conceptual understanding and attitudinal change.

As a trainer I moved beyond explaining and urging. I created a concrete experience for my colleagues, had them reflect on the experience and make their learnings explicit, and then let them make their own way to higher conceptual awareness and a firm commitment to change. The techniques supplied the concrete experience that made deep learning possible.

A conceptual framework that is helpful for understanding this process is participatory learning and action.

Participatory Learning and Action: A Conceptual Framework for Community-based Training

PLA guides my work as a community development advisor to my colleagues, and influences our joint work as trainers of farmers. The core commitments that PLA requires from a trainer are handing over control and initiative to participants, and trusting the participants' abilities (Chambers 2002: 8). These tenets are valued both as a means of achieving desired goals and as ends in themselves. The instrumental value of handing over control and trusting people's abilities takes many forms: high quality data that can be generated by bringing many perspectives to a group process of cross-checking and qualifying and correcting data; deep learning that can result from a group analysis of data; and action plans that are relevant, realistic, and truly supported by the people who will carry them out. The normative value of participatory processes is that they uphold the right of people to be involved in processes that affect their lives (Taylor 2003: 17).

In addition to living participatory values, a trainer who is guided by PLA needs to be a competent technician. The trainer values the knowledge and experience and capacities of the participants, but at the same time brings special expertise to the learning process. This expertise includes: a deep and comprehensive knowledge of the content covered by the training, a sophisticated theoretical understanding of how learning happens and how it can be fostered or impeded, and the technical ability to create catalysts and overcome blocks to learning (Messerli and Abdykaparov 2008: 353). PLA equips trainers with techniques for handing over control and harnessing the creative and analytical abilities of participants. Trainers need to be proficient in using the techniques of the framework. It takes high-level skills in communication, facilitation and conflict negotiation to use a participatory technique successfully (Pretty et al. 1995: 68). An added challenge for the trainer is that true technical proficiency demands much more than the ability to use a technique in isolation. The trainer must also be able to choose the right technique or the right sequence of techniques for the situation (Pretty et al. 1995: 68). To be a competent PLA trainer is to be prepared to adapt or combine techniques or to create new ones, and to be ever mindful of the larger purpose the techniques are designed to serve.

The PLA framework is useful to me because it reminds me of my core commitments as a community development worker. It challenges me to bridge the gap between my espoused values and my values in practice. It provides me with a conceptual way of structuring a learning process: using a participatory technique to create a concrete experience for participants; moving to reflection on the experience to find out what it means and what general learnings can be drawn from it; and creating a space to consider actions that put the learnings to use. This process is depicted in Figure 10.1.

For my Khmer colleagues, the framework is useful because it gives them the tools to challenge the anti-participatory attitudes and behaviours that predominate in a culture with vast divides in social status. It offers a practical alternative to

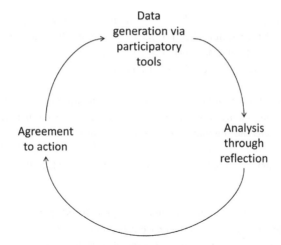

Figure 10.1   The participatory learning and action model

the rote learning and the authoritarian decision-making they are used to in their education system and in their professional lives. It emboldens them to try techniques they had already heard of and were vaguely familiar with, such as role play and visual exercises, but lacked the confidence and technical proficiency to use.

The main limitation of PLA is the risk of techniques being applied mechanically, without living the philosophy behind the techniques, and without achieving the deep learning and the purposeful action the techniques are for. The risk of superficial technique-centred PLA is real in a development industry where demand for training in PLA greatly exceeds the supply of high quality trainers (Chambers 2005: 129–30). A second, related limitation is that the framework lacks a neat, compelling, well-known schematic to highlight that it is a process, not just a toolkit of techniques. David Kolb's (1984) experiential learning cycle is easier to grasp as a process than PLA, which is vulnerable to coming across as a cookbook of exercises rather than a coherent framework for structuring a learning process. How to deal with these limitations is the subject of my concluding reflection.

From Controlling Outcomes to Trusting the Process: Letting go of my own Needs

I used to fret that my colleagues focused too much on the techniques, and not enough on the philosophy of participatory learning and action. I assumed they were reducing the framework to a cookbook of exercises because they did not articulate their practice in abstract terms, as I would. A recent story from my colleagues' training practice exposed the flaws in my assumption.

Two months after we finished our 20 workshops about commune councils, two of my colleagues, Kakada and Saoyan, were contracted by a Cambodian

microfinance institution to provide pig-raising training to two groups of borrowers. I was working in Srer Khmer's head office in Phnom Penh at the time and therefore had no part in creating and delivering this training.
Here is a part of what Kakada told me afterwards:

> In the days before the training, when I was driving my moto or lying in bed, I thought about the methods we used in our workshops about the relationship between citizens and commune councils. For the pig-raising training I wanted to keep the same objective: participants are active. But I asked myself, 'What can I do? What can I change?' I wanted to change the methods to fit this different training ...

> I needed to teach the farmers how to choose good breeding pigs. I divided the farmers into small groups and had each group draw a picture of a pig. I gave everyone a marker pen and asked every member of the group to draw a part of the pig. The farmers enjoyed drawing the pig together and laughed a lot. When the pictures were drawn I had the whole group examine each small group's picture. I explained the content by emphasising with a marker pen the features you need to look for in a good breeding pig ... I changed the parts of the pictures that differed from what a good breeding pig looks like. For example, if the pig in the picture had a curved back I would draw a straight back, and then explain the point ...

Here is a part of Saoyan's story:

> To teach the features of good breeding pigs I formed small groups and asked each group to draw a picture of what they think a good breeding pig looks like. Unlike Kakada I am not good at drawing, so instead of making changes to the drawings I gave each group a photo of a good breeding pig and asked them to spot the differences between their drawing and the photo. Then I explained the content of the session.

> At the end of the training I divided the participants into two groups. I asked the first group to prepare and perform a short play that shows how they raise pigs now. The second group needed to show how to raise pigs using the techniques we covered in the course ... After the performances I asked reflection questions such as: What differences do you notice between the two scenarios? What feelings did this exercise bring up for you?

> That is how I checked the participants' understanding of the content and their level of motivation to use it.

My colleagues took the techniques from our workshops about commune councils and applied them in an original way to a workshop about pig-raising. They created something. They thought for themselves. How did they reach that point?

In the earlier workshops about commune councils, my presence was crucial. I guided my colleagues through their first rehearsal and discussion of the techniques in the office; I was there during their field testing of the techniques in the first few workshops; I led their reflection and analysis of the first few workshops and their refinement of the workshop design as we went along; I ran a series of story-telling sessions after all 20 workshops were finished to help them name their own learnings from the whole experience; and finally, with guidance and encouragement from me, they created and ran a one-day workshop for the whole NGO to share part of what they learned. If none of that had happened – if I had just shown them the techniques over one or two days and left them to it – they would be using the techniques in a superficial and disempowering way today.

My long-term and close presence – as an advisor, a coach, an appreciative friend *and* a critical friend – made it possible for my colleagues to recognise the power of the techniques. I didn't let them use the techniques as a substitute for thought. I introduced them to the techniques through a process that I designed and led with care – a process that ensured they were doing some hard intellectual work every step of the way.

My Khmer colleagues do not describe their learning in the way that I describe mine. I would talk more about enhancing group dynamics, engaging different learning styles, creating chances for skill development and attitudinal change and other such concepts that have meaning for me. My educational and social experiences make those concepts important to me. I would talk less about the techniques themselves. My mistake was to forget that, although I started and nurtured a learning process for my colleagues, I cannot and should not control how they make sense of that process. My colleagues get more excited by the techniques than I do because for them these are revolutionary techniques. These techniques challenge everything they have experienced in their education system and their society. For me these techniques are nothing special because I have experienced them my whole life.

My colleagues' focus on the techniques – a focus that at times seemed unhealthy to me – was not a sign of superficial learning on their part. Learning the techniques made it possible for them to learn something deeper. The techniques convinced them that farmers can do creative and analytical tasks. The techniques extended their own creative and analytical abilities and gave them the confidence to use those abilities in different situations, without my presence. The techniques gave them a completely different perspective on what training can be like for participants: fun, interactive, practical. The techniques changed their view of what designing and facilitating a training event demands from trainers: creativity, thought, teamwork.

My colleagues made sense of their experience in their own way; they made the techniques their own. Their training practice is more creative and more thoughtful as a result, and that's what matters. What doesn't matter is whether they care as much as I do about the analytic distinction between philosophy and techniques. They will never enjoy a philosophical discussion as much as I do, but that doesn't matter either.

Techniques have the power to transform training practice if they are introduced through a months-long process that blazes with creativity, simmers with thought, and sizzles with teamwork.

References

Chambers, R. 2002. *Participatory Workshops: A Sourcebook of 21 Sets of Ideas and Activities*. London: Earthscan.

Chambers, R. 2005. *Ideas for Development*. London: Earthscan.

Kolb, D.A. 1984. *Experiential Learning: Experience as the Source of Learning and Development*. Englewood Cliffs: Prentice Hall.

Messerli, S. and Abdykaparov, M. 2008. Participatory approaches in developing farmer education and community ownership of training in Kyrgyzstan, *Community Development Journal*, 43(3): 358–70.

Pretty, J.N., Guijt, Ir., Scoones, I. and Thompson, J. 1995. *A Trainer's Guide for Participatory Learning and Action*. London: International Institute for Environment and Development.

Taylor, P. 2003. *How to Design a Training Course: A Guide to Participatory Curriculum Development*. London: Continuum International Publishing Group.

Chapter 11

Visiting Memories Together: The Use of a Collective Narrative Pedagogy in Srebrenica

David Denborough

In collaboration with: Sanela Ustic, Ivana Mrvica, Edina Secovic, Mirjana Petrov, Ajla Selimadzovic, Mirela Badurna, Sanela Ahmed, Kristin Windels, Anne van den Ouwelant, Susan Shaw, Laurence Christiaens, Fahir Cimic, Emina Mehic, Mirjana Bunijevac-Petrovic, Johan Van de Putte, Matthias Deleu, Christiaan Deleu, Sam Schurg, Thomas Deleu, Wieke van Belle. The work described in this chapter was a partnership between Crea Thera[1] and Dulwich Centre Foundation International.[2] The training team consisted of David Denborough, Susan Shaw and Johan van Putte.

Wars fought in the territory of the former republic of Yugoslavia, between 1991 and 1995, resulted in the deaths of more than 130,000 people. These were Europe's deadliest conflicts since WWII. This chapter focuses on those who are responding to the aftermath of a specific event in Srebrenica during the Bosnian War. In July 1995, more than 8,000 Bosnian Muslim men and boys were killed in Srebrenica by units of the Army of Republika Srpska (Bosnian Serbs). A further 25,000–30,000 women, children and elderly were forced to flee the Srebrenica area. Two years earlier, in April 1993, the United Nations (UN) had declared the besieged enclave of Srebrenica a 'safe area' under UN protection. However, in July 1995 the United Nations Protection Force, represented by 400 Dutch peacekeepers, failed to prevent the town's capture and the subsequent massacre. The International Criminal Tribunal for the former Yugoslavia, located in The Hague, ruled that the massacre of the Srebrenica enclave's male inhabitants, accompanied by the forcible transfer of all of the women, children and elderly, constituted a crime of genocide. The workshop described in this chapter was attended by Bosnian Muslim and Bosnian

---

1 Crea Thera International is an organization based in Srebrenica which offers creative therapies to the citizens and the society of Srebrenica. For more information, see: www.creathera.com

2 For more information about the work of Dulwich Centre Foundation International see: www.dulwichcentre.com.au/dulwich-centre-foundation.html

Serb practitioners as well as participants from the Netherlands, Belgium, USA and Australia.

The effects of the massacre that took place in Srebrenica in July 1995 continue to influence the lives of local residents. In 2010, fifteen years on, an organisation based in Srebrenica, Crea Thera, approached Dulwich Centre Foundation International requesting a one-week training programme for local practitioners. It was hoped that this training programme, focusing on 'collective narrative practices to respond to trauma/hardship' would assist local people and practitioners in their work, particularly with women and children.

It was only the evening before the workshop was to begin, while sitting in a coffee shop in Sarajevo, that I learned three important pieces of information. Firstly, that both Bosnian Muslim and Bosnian Serb practitioners would be attending the training, as would a number of international practitioners including representatives from the Netherlands, which was the country whose peacekeepers were stationed in Srebrenica during the massacre. Secondly, that the organisers had never before held an event which practitioners from different sides of the conflict had attended. And thirdly, that the workshop would begin with a visit to the Srebrenica – Potočari Memorial Centre and Cemetery for the Victims of the 1995 Genocide.

I can still vividly recall the surroundings of that coffee shop in Sarajevo where I learned these three pieces of information! Fortunately, we then had quite a drive to get to Srebrenica. As the van wove its way through the Bosnian landscape, there was a lot to consider.

Collective narrative practices have been used in a wide range of countries and contexts to respond to individuals, groups and communities who have experienced significant trauma (Denborough 2008, Denborough, White and Wingard 2009, Denborough 2010). This includes contexts in which community members are responding to the horrors of war, occupation, genocide and dispossession. I was prepared for the fact that participants in this workshop and their families may have experienced war, killings, loss, grief and profound hardship.

What I was not prepared for, however, was what it might mean to have people with very different experiences of these events of war be present in the same training programme, particularly if the week was to begin with an immersion in history – namely the visit to the Memorial Centre which honours the victims of the genocide.

While there are a number of examples of narrative therapy principles (White and Epston 1990, White 2007) being applied to 'mediation' and 'conflict resolution' (Winslade and Monk 2000), I had no previous direct experiences as a facilitator/ trainer to draw upon to respond to this particular situation. The use of narrative practices within the realms of 'peace-building' (Lederach 1995), 'reconciliation', 'social healing' (Lederach and Lederach 2010), 'living side by side' (Denborough et al. 2012) are not significantly developed.

This chapter focuses on the challenge of this workshop and how we as trainers and participants collectively responded to it. It describes how we created a collective narrative document during the week, how this was 'performed'/re-told, and what this made possible. Throughout this chapter, I will also theorise about how this process of generating collective narrative documents and convening definitional ceremonies constitutes a particular pedagogy.

Before proceeding, I would like to acknowledge that this was my first visit to Bosnia and to Srebrenica. While the relationships and partnerships formed during this week will continue, this chapter has a modest scope. It focuses simply on how we responded to the challenges and possibilities posed by this one-week training programme which included bridging significant differences.

An Immersion in Memory

As it had already been arranged for workshop participants to visit the Memorial Centre in Potočari, Srebrenica on the first morning, it seemed important to consider how this experience could act as a foundation for our week together. The Memorial Centre powerfully honours all that occurred on that particular site in 1995. Here is a brief description of some of what we witnessed:

> Together we watched a film that conveyed the events that occurred in 1995. We heard from mothers who had been separated at gunpoint from their sons and husbands, and then lost them forever. We saw film footage of refugees, young and old, fleeing and trying to seek sanctuary. We heard of tears flowing like rivers. And we sat in the building where thousands of bodies, which had been excavated from mass graves, were laid in rows before they were reburied. We also visited the 'wall of memory' that lists the names of those killed and we wandered amidst the headstones looking at the ages of those thousands of people whose lives were lost. At times, some of our group members were overcome and had to take some time alone.

Eighteen of us visited the site. Some participants did not visit all the different sections and we did not try to come together to talk about the experience at the site itself. Instead, participants could take all the space and time they needed to wander through the memories of Potočari. We then headed to a local restaurant, sat outside for a time, and shared a meal together. We did not try to discuss as a group what we had seen at the Memorial Centre until the afternoon when we returned to our meeting space and sat together in a circle. To shape this discussion, I offered participants the following invitation:

> Please consider what was particularly important for you in visiting the Memorial site this morning. What aspect of your time there do you wish to carry with you throughout this week? This may relate to a particular image, thought, or memory that was sparked. The visit to the Memorial centre might have confirmed a commitment you have, an obligation that you carry with you. This might be

linked to the work that you are doing. Please turn to the person next to you and discuss whatever it was that was most important to you about the visit, and why it is important to you to carry this with you throughout our meeting this week. Of course, there may also be memories that arose, thoughts you had, that you do not want to remain with you, that you wish to forget. At this time, please focus on those images, ideas or thoughts, that you want to carry with you, and why these are important to you.

While participants were conversing in pairs, the facilitators (Susan Shaw, Johan van Putte and I) took care to listen in, sit with the pairings, and at times assist people to find words that would adequately convey the meanings they wished to share with others. When it came time for participants to speak these to the larger group, translation was required. Participants spoke Bosnian, Dutch, English, and Flemish, so at times three-way translations were required. Facilitators offered their responses alongside participants.

A key aspect of narrative practice involves 'rescuing the said from the saying of it' (Geertz 1973, Newman 2008) and 'translating' the spoken word into written documents that can then be read and performed. Permission was therefore sought by the facilitators to take notes while participants were speaking. Overnight, a document was created from participants' words. I have included extracts from this document called 'Visiting memories together'[3] here.

Visiting Memories Together

Today we met in Srebrenica. We are a group of practitioners from Bosnia, from the Netherlands, from Belgium, from the USA and Australia. This morning, we all headed to Potočari to visit the Genocide Memorial. This is located at the site where Dutch peacekeepers were supposed to create a safe haven for Bosnian refugees, but where instead the greatest massacre in Europe since World War II took place.

We are a group of people from many different perspectives. We speak in different languages. But we all found the experience of being together at the Memorial highly significant. When we considered what was particularly important to us in visiting the Memorial site, and what we wish to carry with us throughout this week, here is some of what we said.

A STRONG IMPULSE TO LIVE AND TO SURVIVE
I am from Bosnia. I was a child during the war and as I was visiting the Memorial, it was as if sharp objects were inside my chest. I was feeling very intensely. Even though I don't have anyone who was killed in Srebrenica, I have the feeling that all the mothers are my mother. All the fathers are my father. And all the children

---

3   If you would like to read the full document I can be contacted at daviddenborough@dulwichcentre.com.au

are me. I cannot understand how this happened. I cannot accept it, but I must hold it and trust that together we can carry it. What I carry with me from today is that I am glad that people from other places are here. We are not only Bosnians here this week and this supports me. It is weird but it is supporting. There is one more thing. Today, after visiting the Memorial, I have such a strong impulse to live and survive in the name of everything that happened here.

SHEDDING TEARS WITH ALL OF YOU RELEASES ME

I would like to speak next because I am from Srebrenica. And today I saw the movie at the Memorial Centre for the first time. The reason why I left the screening, the reason that I was crying so hard, was that we were all looking at the film, but I was seeing different faces. I was seeing the faces of my family who died, those who survived and so on. After a time I just couldn't stand it anymore, I wanted to leave the room. I am glad that I cried. And I am glad that I shared this with all of you. Somehow this releases me, the tears release me, sharing this with you releases me. Now I have the wish to kiss my children, to celebrate that we have life.

HONESTY

Here in Srebrenica, when the UN declared that this region was to become a protected area, everybody was happy. They cheered. They rejoiced that there was going to be safety. But this became a trap. It was not real. I want to keep this memory with me. It will remind me of the importance of honesty, of speaking only what will be followed through, of ensuring that promises do not become traps. This day will remind me of the significance of honesty.

THE STRENGTH OF TRAUMA AND THE STRENGTH OF SURVIVORS

Today, I have a strong image of the opposites of life and death. Love and hope is on one side, and cruelty and murder is on the other side. I see the picture of the boy on a wall crying and holding himself. This is what I remember most strongly. It is an image that brings admiration for those who have survived it all. I have worked for many years here in Bosnia with children and trauma. On one side, I feel the strength of the trauma as pain. On the other hand, I feel the strength of those who survive, who find life again. I want to carry both these sentiments with me.

NEVER AGAIN

My heart is thumping because I went through the war here in this country and I lost many people who I cared about. It is also thumping because during that time I lost all my friendships with Muslims and Serbs. For a time it was impossible to be friends across the divisions. Now we are trying again. Through these five days, I want to go only with one thought: 'never again'. With the help of the younger generation we must learn not to hate each other. I work with children with special needs – Serbs, Croats and Bosnians. I make no distinctions. All of these are like my children. Let us work to ensure 'never again'.

UNDERSTANDING THE 'OTHER SIDE'

My heart is also beating fast and it is very hard to speak, because all this time I was also on the 'other side'. Regardless of that, I feel with people who survived all that happened here. It was especially touching watching when mothers were saying goodbye to their children and husbands. I was putting myself in their place, trying to understand. I'm glad that I am here now so I can try to understand more how it was on that other side. It is important for me. Since I was small, I lived with only one story, now I am here to understand the stories of others.

TO BE AWARE THAT WE COULD BE ON THE SIDE OF DOING GREAT HARM

When I was 11, growing up in Belgium, I read a book written by a Jewish man about how he survived Treblinka. The book changed my life. It made me realise I couldn't be sure that I would never end up on the wrong side. Morally, it made me think that one day I might end up being on the side of doing great harm to others. So back then, when I was 11, I committed to really try to always stay aware of this and to do all I could not to participate in doing harm. Today I felt again this awareness and this commitment. I want to carry this through this week and into the future.

RECOGNISING EACH OTHER

My heart is beating loudly and I need to speak in my language about this. I am from this country and was a refugee during the war. Somehow today was very important to me because we are so mixed here. In the film, there were Dutch people on the screen – the peacekeepers who did not keep the peace – and there are Dutch people here today. We are all watching the suffering of others together. When I go to the Memorial Centre I always talk to those dead people. I always say, I can see you. It is as if I go through a hard difficult cloud, but after talking with them I always come out again and see life. We don't know what the future brings, but I don't want this to ever happen again to my country. I love so much this country and the people in it. Today I see that by living together, by recognising and seeing each other, as we are doing now, there is a way it will never happen again. We must continue to do this.

EXTENDING THE CIRCLES

The stories that we heard, the pictures we saw today, I can link them all to my story. They are the stories of my people, my family. After today, though, I am wondering whether I should also visit the sites where the so-called 'other side' commemorate their victims. Not to belittle or lessen what we have seen in the Memorial today but in order to widen the picture, to extend the circle. I am afraid that our country is still dealing with the divisions that we went through before and that led to the war. I believe that extending the circle might be a way to make a real breakthrough in recognition. This is what I will carry with me this week.

REALISING THE EFFECTS OF THE WAR ON MY LIFE

Watching the movie reminded me of my childhood during the war. I started crying when I saw the mother saying goodbye to her son. It made me remember saying goodbye to my father during the war. I will never be the same after being here in Srebrenica. That's a good thing. After I cry for a while, I am going to understand so much better the pain of the people. And by understanding the suffering here, it helps me to realise more what I went through as a refugee, what my family and everyone around me endured. This is a good thing.

THE RESPONSIBILITIES OF THOSE OF OTHER NATIONS

I did not know that Srebrenica was the world's first UN 'safe protected area'. To think that such a massacre could then take place here is profoundly shocking to me. My country is a part of the United Nations. This makes me think about the responsibilities that my country and every country has in supporting the people of Bosnia and Srebrenica now, to play some part in responding to the injustice of this situation.

ACTS OF CARE AND LOVE IN THE MIDST OF HORROR

What was most significant to me during the film and Memorial, were the acts of love, bravery and care that people were taking in the midst of horror. The men carrying each other as they fled through tracks through the hills, the tears being shed for loved ones' lost, and the mothers' love for their children. There were also the glimpses of what people have been doing since the genocide. The tireless efforts of women trying to find ways to bury their loved ones, the ways in which people are still dreaming of those who have passed away, and how they are carrying on their memories. These acts were all very significant to me. In amidst the greatest horrors, when human beings are treating others with such hatred, there are also acts of care, acts of love. I want to remember this throughout this week. I want to remember not only the horror that happened here in Srebrenica, but also the love of mothers, the images of men trying to carry each other to safety.

There are 18 of us here, from Bosnia and from different countries. This morning we visited memories together. We shared the memories of this place, Srebrenica. Now, we are trying to create something together, and to find ways to support future generations.

The next morning, we (the facilitators) read this document back to the participants. In doing so, we were clear that what we were reading was a draft and we sought participants' feedback as to whether we needed to make any changes to the text. This initial re-telling served two purposes. On the one hand, it involved a collective protocol, inviting each individual and the group, to participate in determining if/ how this document could 'speak for' and represent them. On the other hand, this initial re-telling was a ritual 'performance' (Denzin 2003) in itself, a 'definitional ceremony' (Myerhoff 1982, White 1999) that wove together disparate stories, histories, values and commitments in particular ways.

When this document was read back to those whose words, knowledges, hopes and commitments it represents, it was listened to and responded to as if it was a familiar and treasured piece of music. Participants accompanied the rhythm of the re-telling with nods and gestures. The quiet in the room during the spaces between each theme took on the special quality that is apparent during musical recitals when silence is recognised as equally important as any note. When it came time for participants to give their spoken feedback, they described the document as a faithful representation of their words. More so, they spoke with appreciation of how it had encapsulated the spirit of the day and they requested it be translated into their respective languages so that they could share it with others. Participants were also intrigued by the narrative practices that had been used within the process and were interested in how these could be put to work in their contexts. Significantly, the experience of 'Visiting memories together', which could have led to division, disquiet and fragmentation within the group, had instead contributed to a foundation for further learning and action together. It was as if a 'rich textual heritage' (Lowenthal in Wertsch 2002: 62) was now available to us as a group to build upon.

Reflection

There are two key narrative pedagogical concepts I wish to mention here in relation to the creation and performance of this collective document:

- the invention of unity in diversity
- creating opportunities for resonance.

The Invention of Unity in Diversity

The generation and performance of this document is an example of what Paulo Freire described as 'the invention of unity in diversity' (1994: 157). The introduction and closing statement clearly frame the document collectively: 'This morning we visited memories together. We shared the memories of this place, Srebrenica. Now, we are trying to create something together, and to find ways to support future generations.' And yet the document is constructed through diversity. Other than within the introduction and closing statement, the collective 'we' is used very rarely. Instead, the themes are relayed in the first person and this allows for rich, personal, particular fragments of life and short stories to be shared. Differences of perspective and differences of history are clearly acknowledged within the text. There are very few generalisations offered, and no statements of interpretation about the acts of others. Significantly, words from each participant were 'rescued' (Newman 2008) and included, so that in the re-telling each person recognised their particular contributions. In fact, as the text was read aloud, small unspoken acknowledgements took place between the facilitators and each individual as their words temporarily took centre stage before dissolving back into a collective ethos.

Creating Opportunities for Resonance

The ways in which participants embraced the document 'Visiting Memories Together' indicated that it resonated with them in significant ways. I believe that two different forms of resonance were in play during the production and performance of this collective document:

- a resonance between the text and participants' own experiences, and
- a resonance between one's own stories and the storylines of others.

Creating Opportunities for Resonance between the Text and Participants'
Own Experiences.

The visit to the Memorial Centre evoked a myriad of responses and reverberations for each of us regardless of our social location. The very material we were working with was powerfully evocative. Even so, great care was required in how participants' spoken word responses were 'rescued' and re-presented in a written form, according to particular themes. Within this process, 'rich' or 'thick descriptions' (Geertz 1973) of experience were generated through:

- ensuring that individual's own words (as opposed to facilitators' interpretations or imaginations) were recorded – this is a process of eliciting and re-valuing local knowledge.
- The evocation of particular visual imagery, 'I see the picture of the boy on a wall crying and holding himself.'
- the use of metaphor, '... as I was visiting the Memorial it was as if sharp objects were inside my chest' and,
- the inclusion of sensory description, 'My heart is thumping .. '.

Resonance can be described as a sensory and even artistic experience. The use of participants' exact words and phrases, visual imagery, metaphor and sensory description are therefore likely to increase the possibilities of resonance and reverberation (see White 2006, 2011).

Equally significant in terms of generating rich descriptions is the fact that within the themes, participants link what was significant to them about their experience at the Memorial to their own personal and collective histories. The social histories that explain why a certain experience at the Memorial was meaningful to them are clearly articulated:

'I am from Bosnia. I was a child during the war ... All the fathers are my father.
And all the children are me.'

'I started crying when I saw the mother saying goodbye to her son. It made me remember saying goodbye to my father during the war.'

'My heart is also beating fast and it is very hard to speak, because all this time I was also on the "other side"'.

These linkages across time provide the document with its narrative power. These linkages produce what can be called a 'richly storied text'. When participants heard back their own words and expressions in the collective ritual re-telling of the document, a form of resonance occurred between the text and their own experiences of life:

> [At times when we] … experience the phenomena of reverberation and resonance – the images and themes associated with this inner language have the potential to set off reverberations that reach into the history of our lived experience, and, in response to these reverberations, we experience the resonance of specific memories of our past. These memories light up, are often powerfully visualised, and are taken into the personal storylines of our lives, resulting in a heightened sense of myself (White 2006: 84).

Significantly, the text 'Visiting memories together' is richly storied in ways that also create opportunities for resonance between different people's storylines.

Creating Opportunities for Resonance Between One's Own Stories and the Storylines of Others.

A second form of resonance involves how the storylines of different people(s) relate to one another. The document 'Visiting memories together' has as a key theme the enquiry: What do we want to carry forth from the past into the future? This enquiry invited participants to speak of specific purposes, prized values, hopes and dreams, vows and commitments. These included:

> '[I wish] to remember not only the horror that happened here in Srebrenica, but also the love of mothers, the images of men trying to carry each other to safety.'

> 'I have such a strong impulse to live and survive in the name of everything that happened here.'

> 'Since I was small, I lived with only one story, now I am here to understand the stories of others.'

> 'On one side, I feel the strength of the trauma as pain. On the other hand, I feel the strength of those who survive, who find life again. I want to carry both these sentiments with me.'

Because we had all shared the experience of visiting the Memorial together, and because the document provided rich descriptions of people's particular purposes, values, and hopes, the re-telling of the document provided many opportunities for listeners to place themselves inside the stories of others. Additionally, there were many opportunities for the storylines of participants to intersect with the storylines of others.

The richer, or thicker, the storylines that are developed within a collective document, the more likely it is that some aspect of these storylines will intersect with the storylines of others. This in turn means more opportunities for resonance: more opportunities for the storylines of different people to be brought into relationships of harmony.

I use the musical metaphor of 'harmony' deliberately here. Within pieces of music, harmony is created through the relationship between different melody lines. There can be no harmony if there is only one melody line. During the creation of the document 'Visiting memories together' the hope was not to create similarity or to deny difference, but instead to create opportunities for resonance around what it is that people give value to.

When the document was then performed/re-told to the group, not only did participants experience resonance between the text and their own experience (resulting in a 'heightened sense of [themselves]' White 2006: 84), there were also opportunities for resonance *between* the storylines of participants. This second form of resonance contributed to a heightened sense of 'communitas': a particular form of connectedness that preserves individual distinctiveness (Turner 1969).

A Collective Narrative Pedagogy

This chapter has provided an example of a collective narrative pedagogy put to use in a context in which workshop participants represented diverse histories in relation to an historic conflict. The methodology of collective documentation and the use of a definitional ceremony was 'taught' and simultaneously experienced. This process included:

- inviting participants to richly describe in the spoken and written word what it was they wished to carry forward from their visit to the Memorial site, and why they wished to carry this forward
- collectively documenting and performing this material in ways that contributed to a sense of unity in diversity, and in ways that provided the opportunity for resonance across different storylines.

This particular engagement with history provided a foundation for the rest of the workshop. It also provided examples of particular collective narrative methodologies that participants could put to use in their own contexts.

A Broader Purpose

It seems important to re-iterate that the reason we were meeting in Srebrenica was in order for practitioners to gather new ideas in relation to narrative practice to assist in their work with local women and children who are struggling with social hardships.[4] 'Reconciliation' or 'peace-building' were *not* our primary purpose. Instead, we were united in a wish to contribute to the lives of others in our respective communities, particularly those enduring significant social suffering. This was the common ground on which we stood.

Within collective narrative practice (Denborough 2008) we consistently seek to enable those with whom we are working to make contributions to the lives of others. To be so positioned, no matter the hardships one has endured, is to stand outside passive concepts of victimhood.

As we generated the document included in this chapter, we were doing so with an explicit broader hope. We hoped that this document and the ideas we were exploring might be of relevance to others who are living, working and/or teaching in sites of historic conflict.

References

Denborough, D. 2008. *Collective Narrative Practice: Responding to Individuals, Groups and Communities who have Experienced Trauma*. Adelaide: Dulwich Centre Publications.

Denborough, D. 2010. *Working with Memory in the Shadow of Genocide: The Narrative Practices of Ibuka Trauma Counsellors*. Adelaide: Dulwich Centre Foundation International.

Denborough, D., Wingard, B. and White, C. 2009. *Yia Marra: Good Stories that make Spirits Strong, from the People of Ntaria/Hermannsburg*. Adelaide: Dulwich Centre. In *Holocaust Perspectives: A collection of essays on Holocaust and Genocide*, edited by C. Tatz, 497–435. Sydney: UTSePress. Available http://hdl.handle.net/2100/1349

Denborough, D., White, C., Claver, H.I.P., Freedman, J. and Combs, G. 2012. Responding to genocide: local knowledge and counterstories from genocide survivors in Rwanda, in *Holocaust Perspectives* edited by C. Tatz.

Denzin, N. 2003. *Performance Ethnography: Critical Pedagogy and the Politics of Culture*. Thousand Oaks: Sage Publications.

Freire, P. 1994. *Pedagogy of Hope: Reliving Pedagogy of the Oppressed*. New York: Continuum.

---

4   Collective narrative methodologies that were shared during the remaining training included the Tree of Life, the Team of Life, collective documentation and externalizing conversations (see Denborough: 2008).

Geertz, C. 1973. *The Interpretation of Cultures: Selected Essays*. New York: Basic Books.

Lederach, J.P. 1995. *Preparing for Peace: Conflict Transformation Across Cultures*. Syracuse: Syracuse University Press.

Lederach, J.P. and Lederach, A.J. 2010. *When Blood and Bones Cry Out: Journeys Through the Soundscape of Healing and Reconciliation*. Brisbane: University of Queensland Press.

Myerhoff, B. 1982. Life history among the elderly: Performance, visibility, and re-membering, in *A Crack in the Mirror: Reflexive Perspectives in Anthropology*, edited by J. Ruby. Philadelphia: University of Philadelphia Press, 99–117.

Newman, D. 2008 'Rescuing the said from the saying of it': Living documentation in narrative therapy. *The International Journal of Narrative Therapy & Community Work*, 3, 24–34.

Turner, V. 1969. *The Ritual Process: Structure and Anti-Structure*. New York: Aldine Publishing.

Wertsch, J.V. 2002. *Voices of Collective Remembering*. Cambridge: Cambridge University Press.

White, M. 1999. Reflecting-team work as definitional ceremony revisited. *Gecko: A Journal of Deconstruction and Narrative Ideas in Therapeutic Practice*, 1, 55–82.

White, M. 2006. Working with people who are suffering the consequences of multiple trauma: A narrative perspective. In *Trauma: Narrative Responses to Traumatic Experience*, edited by D. Denborough. Adelaide: Dulwich Centre Publications, 25–85.

White, M. 2007. *Maps of Narrative Practice*. New York: W.W. Norton & Company

White, M. 2011. Revaluation and resonance: Narrative responses to traumatic experience, in *Narrative Practice: Continuing the Conversations*, edited by D. Denborough. New York: W.W Norton & Company, 123–34.

White, M. and Epston, D. 1990. *Narrative Means to Therapeutic Ends*. New York: W.W. Norton & Company.

Winslade, J. and Monk, G. 2000. *Narrative Mediation: A New Approach to Conflict Resolution*. San Francisco: Jossey-Bass.

Chapter 12

Bikin Kacau[1] [*untuk kebaikan*]: Solidarity Education for Civil Resistance in West Papua

Alex Rayfield and Rennie Morello

Introducing the Trouble Making

Bikin kacau means to 'stir-up trouble' in Indonesian. *Untuk kebaikan* means 'for good'. *Proyek Merdeka*[2] [Freedom Project] is about stirring-up trouble ... for good. As activist educators our contribution to 'trouble making for good' is solidarity education; co-learning and co-production of knowledge that grows out of, and in-turn reinforces, a commitment to accompany West Papuans[3] as they expand the contours of freedom.

We were invited to begin this work in 2005. Papuan activists asked us to work with them to strengthen civil resistance in West Papua through popular education. We define civil resistance as: organised, unarmed and extra-parliamentary collective action in the pursuit of political and social goals (Sharp 1973, Schock 2005, Stephan and Chenoweth 2008, Roberts and Garton-Ash 2009).

This chapter explores our understandings and experiences of 'solidarity education'. We talk about where we work, what we are trying to do, and what our understanding of solidarity education is. First, we focus on the solidarity dimension of our educational work, then the educational and pedagogical dimensions of our solidarity. Finally, we explore some of the dilemmas of this work.

---

1 Pronounce *Bikin Kacau* like Bee-kin Ca(t)-chow.

2 The project is independent. It is not a proxy of any government, political party, religious organisation, non-government organisation, community-based organisation, or aid and development agency in any country.

3 In this chapter we use the word Papuans to refer to indigenous Papuans living in the western half of the island of New Guinea which is under Indonesian government control. We refer to this territory, or country as West Papua.

The Context: Where do we Work?

West Papua is an occupied country. The drive from Sentani Airport to the capital Jayapura is about fifty kilometres. The police and military posts line the road like omnipresent sentinels: brooding, watching, and at times lashing out in malevolent fury at Papuan dissenters. Even in the most remote village, you will find a military post. The security forces have a presence everywhere from small hamlets deep in the highlands to the cabinets in the parliaments of Jayapura and Sorong. West Papua is the Indonesian Government's longest running separatist conflict.

On one side is the opponent Indonesian state, actively supported by transnational corporations and foreign governments. For their part, Jakarta[4] uses a combination of sealing the province off from international civil society; terror (consisting of widespread torture of arrested and jailed dissidents, targeted repression and random brutalisation); and the provision of material and political incentives to the Papuan elite to fragment and neutralise Papuan dissent. Alongside these measures they employ a strategy of displacing the indigenous population by swamping the province with Indonesian (non-Papuan) migrants. On the other side are the Papuans, with their long history of resistance, but outnumbered and out-gunned; with few international allies, struggling to unify themselves across political fractures, cultural differences and a rugged geography. This is the context in which the Project takes place: militarised occupation; a struggle for self-determination; participants fresh out of prison; an entire people who have a sense that they are struggling against a relentless tide of what many call 'slow-motion genocide'.

Proyek Merdeka: Where did it Come From and What do we do?

Alex has a relationship with the land and people of West Papua that dates back to 1991. In 2005, Alex was invited to attend a clandestine meeting of West Papuan resistance groups. The meeting was organised by Papuan human rights defenders who, frustrated with a narrow human rights agenda, had begun to explore active resistance to the occupation. As the only non-Papuan present, Alex mostly stayed in the background, listening, observing and talking to people. She was also asked to speak to the whole group on nonviolent struggle. Alex recalls:

> As I rose to deliver my presentation, I took a deep breath. I acknowledged the
> Traditional Owners of the land we were staying on. I acknowledged the sweat

---

4   We speak of Jakarta as a single entity as a form of shorthand for the Indonesian Government. However, we recognise that the Indonesian Government is not a monolith. There is conflict and division amongst those in government about how to deal with the 'Papua problem'. Yet at the same time, the overwhelming majority of Indonesian politicians, officials and military leaders are not willing to even entertain the prospect of an independent state in West Papua.

and tears of those in the room, the sacrifice of people who have since passed on. In formal Indonesian I thanked the organisers for the invitation, then with all the courage I could muster, I told those present that 'I don't support independence'.

You could have heard a pin drop. This was a meeting of independence activists and resistance leaders. Many had spent years in jail for their political beliefs. To my left was Richard Yoweni, the leader of the OPM-TPN[5] faction of the north coast, considered by many in the room to be the Supreme Commander of the guerrillas. I don't think I will ever forget his intense gaze on me at that moment. Kelly Kwalik, the legendary guerrilla leader killed by Indonesian troops in December 2009, had sent a representative who was sitting directly in front of me. Several guys from Markus Victoria, a guerrilla base in Papuan New Guinea, sat to my right, arms folded, forebrow furrowed, eyes focused.

'It is not my role to campaign for independence' I said. 'It is up to you as Melanesians living in the land of your ancestors. And while I am committed to standing in solidarity with you in the pursuit of peace with justice, ultimately it is not Australians like me who would pay the political costs for campaigning for independence. It will be people like you. For me as a non-Papuan to argue for independence would be to assume a colonial mantle. I have no right to presume that I can speak on behalf of what you as Papuans want. Instead,' I went on to say, 'I am committed to accompanying you on your journey ...'.

Alex's presentation outlined the theoretical basis of civil resistance and highlighted some key lessons from other nonviolent struggles around the world that might help maximise the potential for success in West Papua. After the meeting, one of the organisers approached her about 'making concrete' some of the ideas discussed in her presentation. The discussion resulted in a plan, which over time has become the basis for *Proyek Merdeka*. Alex invited Rennie to join the project in 2006.

The ultimate purpose of the Project is to support West Papuans to determine their own future, with or without Indonesian rule. Our contribution to this is to develop a network of people who can resource nonviolent peoples' movements through leadership development, education and participatory action research. We work with five constituencies: young people and students, women, customary leaders, religious leaders, and human rights defenders drawn from every Papuan region. In consultation with our Papuan partners, we work with those committed to, or actively seeking to explore nonviolent ways to achieve social and environmental justice goals. That might include working towards independence but is not limited by that goal.

It is also important to state upfront that while we work in partnership with Papuan resistance leaders and groups, we also make our own political choices about whom we work with.

---

5   Organisasi Papua Merdeka – Tentara Pembebasan Nasional (Papuan National Liberation Army).

When deciding whom we work with we are guided by three critical considerations. Firstly, we only work with those actively committed to or wanting to explore nonviolent methods to transforming conflict. Secondly, we seek to work with all groups committed to transforming the conflict. However, we privilege those groups who choose to focus on civil resistance as opposed to other strategies like lobbying elites and negotiation. Thirdly, we are committed to using the workshops to strengthen unity across political, cultural and gender boundaries.

Our Understanding of, and Reflections on, Solidarity Education

So, what do we mean by solidarity education? Activist education is conducted by and with activists, is openly interested in the processes of change-making, and utilises education to create justice-oriented social change (La Rocca and Whelan 2005). *Proyek Merdeka* facilitates activist education in West Papua. What makes it solidarity education is that we are doing it long-term in an embedded way. By embedded, we mean that the Project is slowly becoming a part of the movement that it aims to support.

In some sense, we might have once identified ourselves as outsiders to the movement offering support 'in solidarity'. However, over time the movement has stirred-up trouble for us and our insider-outsider identities. We work in solidarity with Papuan activists in their struggle for self-determination, but we are not Papuan. In this way, we are cultural outsiders. More importantly, while we attempt to share the risks and costs of working for peace and justice in West Papua, we will never pay the same price as Papuan activists. In this way, we are political outsiders. Connected to this is our commitment to non-interference – Papuan activists themselves must determine the strategic direction and tactical choices of the movement. In this way, we are movement outsiders.

But this is not the whole story. We have a moral and political responsibility to support Papuan aspirations for self-determination. We are regional neighbours. Our own country's government, companies and citizens help enable Indonesian occupation. Australia continues to support and benefit politically and economically from the occupation, so we have a responsibility to change this situation. In this sense, we are movement insiders. We are a part of a transnational movement to bring peace, justice, democracy and liberation to West Papua. Papuans and outsiders all need to work on different pieces of the puzzle that make up the occupation.

For us, solidarity education involves at least five elements: knowledge; relationship; common purpose; capacity and pedagogy. In the next section, we briefly describe each of these and then focus the discussion on the fifth element, pedagogy. We explore some of our pedagogical inspirations, and describe and illustrate one in particular, the spiral model of education. We briefly reflect on some of what we have learnt about facilitating activist education in the Papuan cultural context, and discuss three of many dilemmas of doing this work.

Knowledge

Effective solidarity activists need to understand the histories, cultural context, problems and solutions of the movement we aim to support. As activist educators, we also need to understand how those we are working with think change will happen and how they are working towards their goals.

Relationship

We need to build relationships of trust, and be able to communicate and navigate across political, cultural and linguistic differences over the long-term. The effectiveness of our work relies on the quality, diversity and deepening of our relationships.

Common Purpose

In the context of invitation and relationship, a common goal is negotiated and refined over time. If the collaboration is to avoid contributing further to colonisation, our work needs to support self-determination, rather than impede it.

Capacity

Solidarity educators need to negotiate what is expected, and the tangible contribution they will make to the movement through education and training.

Pedagogy

Our practice of solidarity education is shaped by an educational praxis that is experiential, participatory, elicitive, dialogical, relational, emergent, applied, and change orientated. It is experiential and participatory in that theory and concepts are introduced either through supporting reflection on participants' own experience or through designing highly participatory and creative experiences as part of the workshop process. It is elicitive in that knowledge is drawn from participants through reflection and cultural resources available in the setting. It is dialogical because questions are posed to problematise reality, to stimulate critical thinking, and to open up conversations that (on a good day) transform the ways participants understand themselves and their world. It is relational in that we consciously design workshops (and the Project) in ways that not only form a learning community, but also to help create conditions of trust and safety that enable participants to take the kind of risks necessary to learn. Our approach to education is emergent in that we regularly depart from our workshop agenda. We intentionally leave space in a workshop in order to respond to our assessment of what will assist the group to move deeper and further into learning (Lakey 2010: 145–151). Our pedagogy is applied through consciously seeking to develop skills in our workshops that

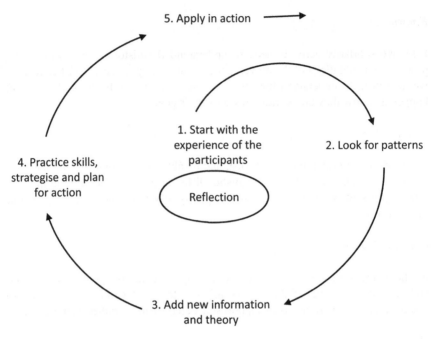

5. Apply in action

4. Practice skills,
strategise and plan
for action

1. Start with the
experience of the
participants

Reflection

2. Look for patterns

3. Add new information
and theory

Source: Used with permission from Rick Arnold, Bev Burke, Carl James, D'Arcy Martin, and Barb Thomas. *Educating for a change*, Toronto: Between the Lines, 1991.

Figure 12.1　The spiral model

support social change as well as creating space for planning action. Finally, our praxis as educators is directed toward enabling collective action for justice, peace and ecological sustainability. Our pedagogy is profoundly shaped by Lakey's (2010) 'direct education', and particularly the 'spiral model' of education which we now discuss.

The spiral model (Arnold et al. 1991, Hammond and Gell 2009) is shown in Figure 12.1 and differs from Kolb's well-known learning model (Kolb 1984) in two respects. Firstly, within the spiral model reflection happens at every stage of the process, as opposed to being a distinct stage. Secondly, the spiral model includes an extra stage that is strategising and planning for action prior to application. So in a sense then, whereas Kolb's model assumes capacities to leap from generalising to application the spiral model takes more care to consider plans for action prior to application/action. The spiral model takes its name from the idea that the learning process takes the shape of a spiral. Each stage leads naturally to the next, and by applying the learning in action (and sometimes in the workshop context), this then generates a new experience, which begins the cycle again. In this way, learning can be taken to a new level, spiralling upwards.

When we design and facilitate education, we use the spiral model to inform the design of each separate session and the design of the entire workshop. For example, a multi-day workshop can take the following format:

- Stage One: Reflecting on participants' experience of civil resistance.
- Stage Two: Look for and draw out patterns or common experiences.
- Stage Three: Elicit theoretical concepts from the group or share generalised knowledge or other examples of civil resistance.
- Stage Four: Apply that new information to the experience of participants and consider new ways of organising civil resistance in their context.
- Stage Five: Conclude the workshop with strategies and action plans for people to apply when they leave.

Throughout all these stages we support reflection. We use a mixture of learning methodologies from all four learning channels: visual, audio, kinaesthetic and emotional. A stage might involve only one exercise or it might include several different learning processes that build on one another. At the same time, each one of these processes progressively moves the five stages of the spiral model.

For example, in a workshop session on applying strategy skills, we might invite participants to share metaphors through talking, drawing, drama, or even body-sculptures (stage one). One Papuan uses metaphor to describe strategy in this way:

> I am a Highlander. So for me desiring freedom is like wanting to eat a banana. In the Highlands, if you want to eat a banana you have to begin at least six months before. You have to clear land for a garden. You must nourish the soil. You need a fence so the garden is not destroyed by animals. You have to find a banana sucker; plant it, water it, care for it, make sure it's not overcome by weeds. Only when the banana plant has grown and the fruit has been harvested do you get to eat it. It is the same with *merdeka* [freedom]. We Papuans need a strategy; we need a plan. We have to think long-term. We must plant and care for a garden now if we want to eat the fruit tomorrow.

Others might use the image of a soccer game or the metaphor of a long fishing trip to illustrate the meaning of strategy. These meaning-rich 'codes' become doors to unpacking Papuan knowledge about strategy and move the group toward developing shared understandings (stage two). If needed, and in the context of a facilitated discussion we might add our own understanding of strategy or reflect on examples from other case studies we have learnt about (stage three). By building on shared understandings and experiences, we are able to review and analyse movement strategy or apply new processes for developing strategy (stage four). One of the tools we like to use in a stage four strategy learning process is the critical path exercise.

Critical path analysis is a tool developed by the Change Agency.[6] In this exercise, participants imagine a world where their vision for change is broken down into something achievable in the next three, five or ten years. Participants then consider the changes required to manifest this vision as a series of outcomes that fall like dominoes towards their vision. We usually map these steps out on paper plates so that the outcomes are recorded. Each specific outcome that logically leads towards the goal is written on a separate paper plate. The plates are arranged like stepping-stones across a river that can be shuffled around in a different order. We ask participants to start by writing their vision as a goal and then work backwards, recording a series of changes or outcomes right back to the present time. By establishing the changes that participants think are required, and the order in which they think these changes need to occur, participants can start identifying the specific objectives their campaigns need to work towards. When participants start to talk about tactics (which activists nearly always do) we ask them to write the tactics down that they believe will achieve the specific outcome on the flip-side of the plate. In this way, the exercise stays outcome-focused. It supports participants to plan for success rather than think in terms of random and isolated tactics.

In one workshop participants took the paper plates home. They used them to explain and discuss their strategy with other activists who had not participated in the workshop (stage five). We met one of these activists a year after a workshop we had facilitated. He told us that after the workshop he returned to his city and facilitated a weeklong workshop with other young activists. Of all the 'tools' he learnt he felt the *jalan ke sukses* ['critical path' in Indonesian, or road to success] was most helpful because it helped people from different perspectives to start talking. He told us it was especially useful as a way of bringing Highlanders and coastal peoples together. He felt it was important for people to learn that 'if you want to do something big, you have to start with something small.' These kinds of processes 'turn people on fire … it makes them realise it's [achieving *merdeka*] a long process but they can do little things now to get to their final destination.'

The same critical path described above helped influence the movement's decision to occupy the provincial parliament for two days in June 2010. This experience (stage five) then becomes the basis of reflection at a subsequent time (stage one) and so on, following the spiral through stages two to five again. In our experience, the spiral model creates space for Papuans' experience, cultural values and traditions. It honours and builds on a rich reservoir of Papuan knowledge about how to survive and make change. And people tell us it works. Some say the workshops are their first experience of educational processes that liberate rather than domesticate.

In the last five years, we have learnt a lot about pedagogy in the Papuan context. Our own experience has taught us that fun team building kinaesthetic exercises, especially at the start of the workshop, build the container (Lakey 2010).

---

6   http://www.thechangeagency.org. See also Chapter 5 in this volume.

They loosen people up, stimulate laughter, which eases tension and generates trust. We are also learning that giving space for people to talk and tell stories is critical. And we lace our descriptions of concepts with metaphors, as well as visual representations. We try to slow down, to facilitate deeper learning. Cultural protocols shape our educational practice. Workshops echo with song. Each day opens and closes with prayer.

Throughout all of this we have also learnt that coordinating a cross-cultural training project for civil resistance in a repressive context, and sustaining relationships of trust across time and space while doing so, is difficult ... very difficult. But we are committed to the long haul. This means systematically working through challenges. In the next section, we describe three of the dilemmas we face and our efforts to manage or overcome them.

Dilemma One: Working Outside Our Own Culture

There are many challenges of doing education outside our own culture. It can bring up a range of issues about our own personal capacity, which in turn impacts on our capacity to engage in solidarity education. Rennie reflects on his experience struggling with this:

> As a relatively experienced activist educator, *Proyek Merdeka* challenges my sense of capacity – deeply. My first opportunity to work with Papuans was a workshop in Papua New Guinea in 2007. I spent the month leading up to the workshop urgently reading all I could about the history, problems and solutions – wanting to make sure I understood the context and issues. This is usual practice for me as an educator – I want to know what I can about the people I am working with, the context in which they are working, what they want to achieve, and how they have been trying to achieve it. I also wanted to understand the different organisations and networks, their relationships with each other, their constituencies and their theories of change. I thought I was ready.
>
> On the first of a ten-day workshop (after days of trouble-shooting a range of logistical challenges, including building showers and toilets for the forty-odd participants), I walked up to the person I was told would be my translator. The workshop was to be held in Indonesian, which I do not speak fluently. I introduced myself, told her how grateful I was for her support. She looked at me blankly. An alarm sounded deep within. I tried again, 'Thank you for agreeing to be my translator; I am looking forward to working with you'. She set me straight. She wouldn't be translating for me; she was not sure where I got that idea from. She was happy to translate from *Tok Pisin* to Bahasa Indonesia (Indonesia's official languge) – which proved helpful because when we work in Papua New Guinea, English is often the third language. But at that moment I felt deeply confronted, I do not speak *Tok Pisin* fluently either. The workshop was

about to begin. I was to lead the opening, introductions, scope the purpose and agenda for the ten days.

As an educator and facilitator, I rely heavily on my senses – seeing, hearing, speaking – reading body language, listening to the intonation in people's voices, their turn of phrase. For me, facilitating in a language that you are not fluent in is like swimming underwater. You cannot really see that well, you cannot hear so well and you definitely cannot speak well. All up, things seem blurry, unclear and otherworldly. Facilitating in this context – underwater – strips me of my usual strengths and capacities and leaves me wondering what I thought I was doing in the name of supporting others.

It is more than four years since that first day and I am still deeply challenged by my capacity to communicate. Sure, there is a practical dimension – just get some good simultaneous translation (which for those of you who are familiar with multilingual environments might agree is not as easy as it sounds). But it is more than that. This disconnect undermines my capacity as an educator, as a solidarity activist. Language is just the beginning of the cultural divide. On so many levels, I am different, an outsider: I cannot help but question what I could possibly offer to a movement of people who are working on such ambitious goals; whose cadre have spent years, sometimes decades in prison; whose leaders are followed, threatened, poisoned and assassinated; and whose constituencies, for the most part, are just trying to survive.

Working across difference as an educator or activist, be it race, culture, class, gender, age or ability is challenging. But it is what active solidarity calls for. As an educator, it is our commitment to co-learning that helps us grapple with these challenges. If it is truly mutual and we are not just learning on other people's time, then it is worth it. We have been invited to make a contribution, and as for all solidarity activists, it is up to us to use our privilege and develop our own personal capacity to step up to the challenges involved in making that contribution. It is important in this context that the Project maintains long-term involvement of our educators, because each opportunity to contribute strengthens our personal and organisational capacity, and therefore strengthens our solidarity education work.

Dilemma Two: Navigating the Tension between Solidarity as Organisers and Solidarity as Educators

As popular educators, we are committed to working with people respectfully, to honour their experiences and to facilitate a space which relies on them making the decisions – it is their campaign, it is their lives. It is never easy to decide when it is legitimate to tell people what we think, what we know, what we would do. We know our rank and power as facilitators often privileges our opinions, even when we say that activists are the experts on their own movement.

In late 2010, we were invited to work with a group of 80 strong-headed activists, the radical margin of the student movement, a group that has close associations with elements of the armed struggle. The mainstream of this group are from remote parts of West Papua known as the Highlands, an area that is significantly disconnected from the global context. After facilitating an edgy discussion about violent versus nonviolent action, and means versus ends, two different people got up, one after the other and told us very clearly that we were outsiders, that they were the movement, and it is Papuans themselves who will win the fight for freedom. We agreed. Then in different ways, both asked what they (the movement) should do. They wanted us to provide an answer, a solution that would solve the Papuan conflict and give them freedom. What issue would generate international attention? Should they kidnap us now? What is the answer? In summary, what we heard these two people say was: 'Don't tell us what to do! Tell us what to do!'

There is an obvious tension here – our commitments to self-determination, non-interference and impartiality have meant that we focus on the process and leave Papuans to make decisions about strategy and tactics. Of course, we interrogate and challenge those decisions in the spirit of robust dialogue, but ultimately it is up to Papuans themselves to plot their own strategic and tactical trajectory. However, the conversation with these activists sharpened the conflict between the educator and solidarity dimensions of our work, that is, between our solidarity as organisers and our solidarity as educators. As educators, we refrain from telling people what to do in favour of challenging participants to think for themselves. But as organisers we could see that these activists' false assumptions about the international community and their own distress of living under a military occupation impairs their ability to analyse the context and make strategic decisions. They need some clear information in order to make their own choices. As organisers, we have a responsibility to share what we know. The problem is that what we know is completely shaped by who we are, what we believe, and how we live. And as educators, we are in a position of power that we do not want to misuse.

As educators, we need to find ways to share information and outside perspectives so that people can make informed strategic decisions. As organisers who have been accompanying the movement for five years (at the time of writing) we now feel there is a role for us to carefully speak to Papuan strategising, but only in the context of strong relationships, invitation and a pedagogical process that starts with experience and reflection, and is directed by questions and listening rather than telling.

Dilemma Three: Funding the Work

On an organisational level the key dilemma this Project faces is finding sustainable funding. Like most activist and community work there is always more that can be done. We would like to write that donors have been quick to recognise the need to fund training and nonviolent efforts to resolve the Pacific's longest running conflict. But this is not the case. Previously, four international non-government organisations (INGOs) have funded the work. All of them have since withdrawn support because they did not want to jeopardise their relationship with the Indonesian government.

The problem, we were told, was not the quality of our work, or the outcomes. Funding agencies claim to value our work; they just do not want to fund it. As one worker expressed in a confidential email to Alex, 'Despite the absolute value we see in the work you are doing on nonviolent transformation [through the Project] we are unable to [continue to] support this initiative financially.' Thus we are left with the sense that there are significant international funders who have decided that it is just too difficult to accompany Papuans in their struggle for justice, even when that struggle is waged through nonviolent means; and resourcing the efforts of those who do is equally as difficult.

By taking this approach, INGOs collude with the Indonesian government's policy of restricting the political space in West Papua. The Indonesian government of course denies this. 'Indonesia still opens its door to [I]NGOs that want to operate in [West] Papua, as long as they benefit the people without involvement in politics and commercial activities' said one government official (The Jakarta Post 2010). Jakarta sees INGOs as 'separatist' trouble-makers but the Indonesian government's continued isolation of the territory just makes it look like they have something to hide.

The reluctance of donor institutions to support social movements in West Papua is ironic. Many INGOs recognise that social movements are fundamental to addressing poverty. Some like Duncan Green (2008) argue that supporting social movements should be INGO core business. But, despite this rhetoric, in our experience INGOs have been reluctant to even find creative backdoor avenues to support citizen organising and mobilisation for justice, rights or peace in West Papua. Many aid and development agency workers we have spoken with are unhappy with these decisions but feel unable to change the risk-adverse culture, which appears to determine decisions.

Perhaps one advantage of the lack of external support is that it helps foster a culture of self-reliance. Papuans need to depend on their own resources rather than external support. It certainly compels us to build a transnational network with stronger, denser and quantitatively more ties. And in the end that is exactly what West Papua needs.

Continuing the Trouble Making

There are risks to all of us when we resist oppression, stand up for liberation and work actively in solidarity. We resist the temptation to retreat into fear – of stirring-up too much trouble for ourselves, for our Project partners, for our families, our funders, or our government. On the other hand, we are mindful that some in both the Australian and Indonesian governments will see our work as unwanted, perhaps even dangerous, foreign intervention. Therefore, we need to be careful. But we also need to ensure we use our privilege ethically. Papuans are being oppressed. Their land is occupied. They have the right to rise up and struggle for freedom. They have the right to invite people to stand up with them and contribute to that struggle. Moreover, it is our privilege (and responsibility) to accompany Papuans on that journey. Solidarity means a willingness to share the costs of political struggle. Solidarity education means doing that through facilitating education designed and directed toward justice.

The reality is, standing with the oppressed and working hand-in-hand for liberation is to *bikin kacau*, to stir-up trouble for yourself, your life and for others, as well as laying some foundations for a more sustainable and just peace. So what does it mean for us, as educators and outsiders, to stoke the fire in someone's belly which is burning for freedom, when as some people have suggested, 'That person could be jailed, shot or worse'? We do not have easy answers. There is incredible tension and uneasiness here. We take responsibility for participants' safety seriously while recognising Papuans' own agency – after all they are already choosing to fight for self-determination nonviolently, and are actively looking for tools and support to do this more effectively. This drives us to actively explore the opportunities to offer support where we can and find a pedagogy that fits.

Like we said, this is to *bikin kacau* … for everyone; hopefully for good.

References

Arnold, R., Burke, B., James, C., D'Arcy, M. and Thomas, B. 1991. *Educating for a Change*. Ontario: Between the Lines.

Green, D. 2008. *From Poverty to Power: How Active Citizens and Effective States Can Change the World*. United Kingdom: Oxfam International.

Hammond, H. and Gell, P. 2009. Exploring praxis: Defining our educational philosophy and making it real, *New Community Quarterly*, 7(4), 28–30.

The Jakarta Post, 2010. Indonesia welcomes Foreign NGOs in Papua. [Online: *West Papua Advocacy Network*, 7 August]. Available at: http://westpapoea. wordpress.com/2010/08/07/indonesia-welcomes-foreign-ngos-in-papua/ [accessed: 1 May 2012].

Kolb, D.A. 1984. *Experiential Learning: Experience as the Source of Learning and Development*. Englewood Cliffs: Prentice Hall.

Lakey, G. 2010. *Facilitating Group Learning: Strategies for Success with Diverse Adult Learners*. San Francisco: Jossey-Bass.

La Rocca, S.E. and Whelan, J.M. 2005. *Activist Education* [Online: The Change Agency]. Available at: http://www.thechangeagency.org/01_cms/details. asp?ID=36. [accessed: 1 February 2011].

Roberts, A. and Ash, T.G. eds 2009. *Civil Resistance & People Power: The Experience of Non-Violent Action from Gandhi to the Present*. Oxford: Oxford University Press,

Schock, K. 2005. *Unarmed Insurrections: People Power Movements in Nondemocracies*. Minneapolis: University of Minnesota Press.

Sharp, G. 1973. *The Politics of Nonviolent Action*. Boston: Peter Sargent Publishers.

Stephan, M.J. and Chenoweth, E. 2008. Why civil resistance works: The strategic logic of nonviolent conflict, *International Security*, 33(1), 7–44.

Chapter 13

Progressive Contextualisation: Developing a Popular Environmental Education Curriculum in the Philippines

Jose Roberto Guevara

'When do we start studying?'

This was the question that was posed to me by a participant after an acquaintance activity that opened the basic awareness to environmental action workshop called RENEW (Restoration Ecology Workshop). The workshop was conducted by the Center for Environmental Concerns – Philippines (CEC-Phils), in partnership with a local federation of sugar workers on the island of Negros, Central Philippines, in the early 1990s.

The acquaintance activity involved participants sitting in a circle, with one participant standing in the middle. The participant in the middle approaches one of the seated participants and introduces himself (all the participants in this particular workshop were men although we did have female and male facilitators). After the exchange of names (often with a handshake) the participant in the middle asks the seated participant, 'What have you done to take care of the environment?' If the response of the seated participants is 'I plant trees', then all seated participants who have also planted trees need to stand up and exchange seats. The person in the middle has to try to grab a seat while the participants are rushing to exchange seats. The participant left standing then has to introduce himself to one of the seated participants and ask what he has done to take care of the environment. After a few rounds of introductions, responses to the question, grabbing seats and laughter, the participants are often energised enough to start the workshop.

It was just after I called an end to the activity that the participant asked me the question, 'When do we start studying?'

I explained to him, 'We already started.'

He looked at his new notebook and pencil that were given to all the participants as part of their workshop kits, then looked up at me very puzzled and went back to his seat in the circle.

I paused.

Then it dawned on me that while I was aware that we had already started studying, the puzzled participant was not aware, or did not even recognise that we were already learning. The empty notebook for me was the sign. Perhaps from his experience studying involves copying something from the blackboard to the notebook or passing knowledge from the teacher to the student. I understood that for him all we had just done was play a game.

I asked everyone to sit down and I approached this participant, 'What was your response when asked, what have you done to take care of the environment?' He replied, 'Save water.' I then went around the circle to ask the other participants for their responses and wrote these on the blackboard. On completing the list of more than twenty environmental actions, I asked, 'Who did not stand up at any time during the activity?' They shouted, 'Everyone stood up, at least once.' This was followed by another participant saying, 'We all do something to take care of our environment.'

With nods around the circle, I said, 'The list of environmental activities you all identified will be what we shall study in this workshop. More specifically, we will get a better understanding of why these actions are important and how we can as individuals and as organisations sustain this level of environmental action.' I then proceeded to explain the topics to be covered by the workshop and the approach we would use. I specifically explained, 'Your active participation in the activities will help facilitate a more participatory approach to learning. This approach acknowledges that we all come with knowledge and experience. It is in the sharing of this knowledge that we are all able to discover and learn new knowledge that we can then apply to our own local environments. This is why the workshop is described as an awareness to environmental action workshop.' At the end of the introductory session, the participant who had earlier asked me the question came up with his now scribbled-on notebook and said, 'Thank you. I now know that we have started to study.'

This incident illustrates a typical moment in the conduct of a community-based training workshop where as facilitators we find the need to adjust the planned activities to respond to the needs of the participants. Some would describe this as an example of being learner-centred, where the workshop design was adjusted to the specific context or situation of the participants. It may seem like a small adjustment, because all I did was to list the actions identified by the participants. But, as this story illustrates, it was this small adjustment that helped establish a link between the acquaintance activity and the workshop objectives and design, and more importantly introduced the participants to the experience of a different way of learning.

However, for me the experience was a big adjustment, because it made me reflect on my own assumptions about the importance of participatory approaches to learning, especially after having been confronted by dominant ways of learning that the workshop's participants were more familiar with. For many of the community-based participants we worked with throughout the 1990s in the Philippines, their main experience of studying would be in a formal school context, where rote learning was the norm, similar to what Paulo Freire (1993) called the 'banking concept of education'. Therefore, the challenge we faced was not merely to develop and implement a grassroots environmental education curriculum to help address the worsening state of the Philippine environment, but to negotiate between our ideals of participatory and empowering environmental education and the realities of the entrenched ways of learning and teaching that our participants and we ourselves had grown up with.

At CEC-Phils, we called this on-going process of adjustment and negotiation, progressive contextualisation. This chapter examines the different ways this educational practice of progressive contextualisation contributed to the development of CEC-Phils grassroots environmental education curriculum.

CEC-Philippines: Responding to the Need for Environmental Education and Action

The CEC-Philippines is an environmental Non-Governmental Development Organisation (NGDO) that has been in operation since 1989. It was established by the national sectoral[1] federations of peasants, fishers, women, indigenous peoples and by a network of NGOs identified with the progressive[2] people's movement in the Philippines after the 1986 People Power Revolution.

It was during this period that the so-called 'democratic space' encouraged the proliferation of NGOs with a wide range of development frameworks. While the socio-political context looked promising, the environmental situation in the Philippines was alarming. A World Bank Country Study (1989: ix) argued that this situation was, 'inextricably bound up with population and poverty problems' and 'closely linked to the problem of unequal access to resources.'

However, despite the mandate and support from the progressive social movement, Noel Duhaylungsod, CEC-Phils first Executive Director noted that in terms of environmental action: ' .. the essence of the task had to be evolved, primarily because environmentalism had little attention from the workers of the social movement for change and development.' (1995: 6).

CEC-Phils initial task was to establish baseline information on the state of the Philippine environment, grounded not solely on statistical data but on stories of communities and individuals directly affected by the declining environmental

---

1   It is important to note that the use of 'sector' in the Philippine context refers to the basic economic sectors of society, namely the workers, peasants, fishers, indigenous peoples, women and so on, which is different from the reference to sectors in Chapter 1 of this book.

2   'Progressive' refers to organisations linked to a particular ideological block within the Philippine political left, who themselves are further divided along ideological and political lines into the 'national democrats (split into several groupings), popular democrats, democratic socialists, and socialist.' (Coronel Ferrer 1997: 5). Aside from its political links, CEC-Phils is also identified with the progressive people's movement because of CEC-Phils focus on grassroots sectors, more specifically the mass-based groups of fishers and peasants (Arquiza 1993: 6).

conditions. In response, CEC-Phils proposed a participatory environmental research framework and distributed this framework to organisations in the 11 sites around the Philippines nominated by the CEC-Phils board members, who themselves held leadership positions within these progressive sectoral federations and organisations.

However, this initial attempt to develop a research framework was met by serious difficulties, 'the most significant [being] the inadequate research capability of our organizations' (Duhaylungsod 1995: 6). This resulted in the identification of grassroots environmental education as the key approach that CEC-Phils would take in working with local communities and organisations.

CEC-Phils called its grassroots environmental education practice popular environmental education, understood as 'an alternative education approach that focuses on the poorer sectors of society, in order to empower them to act collectively within the context of the wider social movement towards liberation.' (Guevara 2002: 43).

CEC-Phils Grassroots Environmental Education Curriculum

The sugar workers in the opening story were attending CEC-Phils Restoration Ecology Workshop which was formulated in 1990 and can be described as the seed workshop from which the entire grassroots environmental education curriculum grew.

As the story illustrates, CEC-Phils was committed to an educational approach that was enjoyable, creative, participatory and empowering. The CEC education workshops were designed with the aim of developing a basic scientific understanding of the environment and how it functioned. The core message is based on the ecosystem concept; that all components of the environment are interconnected and interrelated to each other. Despite this focus in developing a scientific understanding, CEC-Phils workshops challenged the dominant characterisation of environmental problems as technical problems that required scientific solutions. It introduced a holistic analysis where environmental problems were viewed as intricately related to the local socio-economic, political and cultural situation. Furthermore, these local environmental problems were situated within specific sectoral, and broader national and global contexts. And finally, this understanding was meant to inform existing environmental actions (as the acquaintance activity aimed to do), or assist in identifying possible individual and collective environmental actions. Table 13.1 outlines the workshop structure and flow of RENEW.

A core strategy of CEC-Phils educational approach was a commitment to the development of the capacity of local, community-based and sector-based educators, which meant that prior to each basic RENEW workshop, the local organisers attended a RENEW Trainers Training workshop. As well as being a local capacity-building strategy the Training workshops were a response to

Table 13.1   RENEW conceptual learning map matched with RENEW topics

Stages in the RENEW conceptual learning map	Topics
Awareness	acquaintance, release, expectation check and orientation environmental situation (national and global)
Understanding	ecosystem concept ecosystem structure ecosystem function balance of nature environmental situation (national and global)
Action	vision towards environmental action evaluation celebration

Source: Guevara 1995.

CEC-Phils educators who were fluent in only a number of the major languages spoken in the Philippines. At the conclusion of the RENEW Trainers Training, the new facilitators were guided in adapting the workshop programme and design to suit the local context and the nature of the participants, and were mentored as they co-facilitated the workshop.

Out of the basic RENEW workshop grew the rest of the grassroots environmental education curriculum (Figure 13.1). The curriculum consisted of advanced courses that were more problem-specific; skills-based workshops that assisted communities in responding to specific environmental issues; or were adapted to fit the needs of specific sectoral groups. For instance, the Community-based Rehabilitation Technology (CORETECH) workshops were aimed at developing skills to respond to environmental problems like a snail infestation of rice paddies, rehabilitation of volcanic ash, inundated agricultural lands or rehabilitation of damaged coral reefs. The Community-based Environmental Monitoring (CBEM) workshops were aimed at developing skills and processes for monitoring environmental disturbances often caused by industrial pollution while sector-specific workshops were designed for peasants, women, urban poor, fisherfolks and indigenous peoples. Problem-specific and area-based workshops were also designed to familiarise communities with the potential impact of mining or agro-industrial estates on their livelihoods.

CEC-Phils Practice of Progressive Contextualisation

The initial activity that the sugar workers participated in used the game as an acquaintance activity, however, it can be used for other purposes depending on which RENEW module is being conducted. For example, it may be used as part of

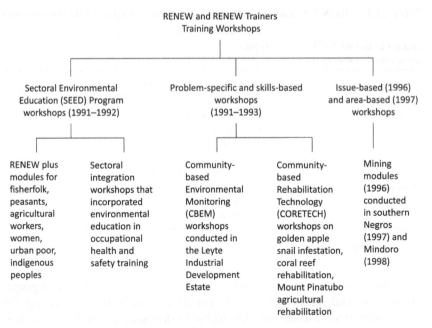

RENEW and RENEW Trainers
Training Workshops

Sectoral Environmental Education (SEED) Program workshops (1991–1992)	Problem-specific and skills-based workshops (1991–1993)	Issue-based (1996) and area-based (1997) workshops

| RENEW plus modules for fisherfolk, peasants, agricultural workers, women, urban poor, indigenous peoples | Sectoral integration workshops that incorporated environmental education in occupational health and safety training | Community-based Environmental Monitoring (CBEM) workshops conducted in the Leyte Industrial Development Estate | Community-based Rehabilitation Technology (CORETECH) workshops on golden apple snail infestation, coral reef rehabilitation, Mount Pinatubo agricultural rehabilitation | Mining modules (1996) conducted in southern Negros (1997) and Mindoro (1998) |

Source: Modified from Duhaylungsod 1998.

Figure 13.1   CEC-Phils grassroots environmental education curriculum

the concluding Vision to Environmental Action module to help identify the need for networking across sectors. In this instance, a different question is used, 'Who do you work with to take care of the environment?'

The educational practice of adjusting an activity[3] to suit a specific purpose and stage within a workshop, and the on-going adaptation, revision and renewal of RENEW was described by Duhaylungsod (1995) as progressive contextualisation. This description is based on the work of Andrew Vayda (1983) who described progressive contextualisation as a methodology in human ecology research that 'involve[s] a focus on significant human activities or people-environment interactions and the explanation of these [interactions] by their placement within progressively wider or denser contexts' (1983: 265).

Because of emphasis in encouraging the newly trained facilitators to adapt the workshop to the local context, CEC-Phils version of progressive contextualisation was primarily described as localisation (Guevara 2002). This process is very

---

3   I first encountered this activity as an icebreaker where the question was about more personal characteristics such as, 'What do you like wearing?', so if you answer 'Sandals', all those wearing sandals stand up and exchange seats. We were keen that even so-called icebreaker activities had an environmental theme and contributed towards achieving the learning objectives of the workshop.

similar to what Freire (1993: 66) described as responding to the 'here and now', in particular 'the situation within which [people] are submerged, from which they emerge, and in which they intervene.'

The following sections will examine the different manifestations of progressive contextualisation that have been identified from CEC-Phils practice. The first section describes progressive contextualisation as localisation; this was the starting point of what we initially viewed to be curriculum development practice. Elements of this localisation approach are examined, including the value of the links between the local and the global in grassroots environmental education. The second section examines progressive contextualisation as an on-going and reciprocal process between curriculum development and the dynamic local and global contexts. It identifies dimensions of this on-going characteristic and argues for a more explicit research agenda that enables this process to become developmental rather than repetitive.

Progressive Contextualisation as Localisation

The key factors that informed the localisation process were the participant's background and the specific environmental situation that prompted the local host organisation to invite CEC-Phil to conduct a RENEW workshop.

The host organisation helped to identify the participants' level of literacy, knowledge, skills and experience, which in turn determined the language and the learning methods to be used. English was used as the base language of RENEW, however, CEC-Phil educators were constrained by their own language limitations when they designed the workshop that relied on key sources of information and knowledge written in English. Language was not so much a problem when conducting the RENEW Trainers Training as most of the educators within the progressive social movement could speak basic English. When participants were not able to understand English, the local facilitators also acted as translators.

What was common across the wide range of participants was the desire for a more active approach to learning. While this seemed easy to design and conduct, the sugar worker's story reminded us of the importance of introducing participants to an active approach to learning given that their experience was more of a classroom-based 'banking' system of learning. Therefore, a more conscious process was required to ensure that key lessons were clearly identified and that the active participation and resulting enjoyment did not overshadow the main learning aim.

While the organisational affiliation of the participants was often a key characteristic that assisted in the process of progressive contextualisation, the specific individual context was often not considered by CEC-Phils educational practice. This was because the participants were usually members of a local people's organisation, a sectoral group, an NGO or a network, and therefore the emphasis was on working with them as a collective rather than as individuals. This tension between the collective and the individual is further demonstrated by the tendency in the 1980s and 1990s for the growing global green movement to focus on individual behaviour change, rather than systemic change, as advocated by the progressive social movement in the Philippines.

However, one can argue that the local, as defined by the individual, primarily remains the significant starting point of any educational process, while acknowledging the value of collective action. Therefore, contextualisation begins with an understanding of one's own position within these wider and denser contexts, and as Freire argues, this is an on-going process that has to be viewed as part of a movement, and that 'The point of departure of the movement lies in the people themselves' (1993: 66).

Aside from the participants, the local was also a particular space (a small community, an entire province, an administrative region or the Philippines) and location of a specific environmental problem. This particular locale, while often spatially or geographically defined, could also be relational, such as a shared characteristic among the participants. For example, it could be a common environmental problem, like a foreign company proposing to establish mining operations in different parts of the country, or a common work identity, like a sectoral group of workers, women, peasants, or indigenous peoples, from different parts of the country.

This practice of progressive contextualisation as localisation is consistent with a key principle of community development identified by Jim Ife (2002: 211) who identifies the importance of 'valuing the local' that includes valuing local knowledge, culture, resources, skills and processes. However, within an environmental context, to have the local as the starting point of contextualisation requires that a connection to the global be simultaneously considered. This is consistent with what the environmental movement has been successful in establishing, the clear connection between the local and the global, as enshrined in the phrase 'Think Local, Act Global.' There is no lack of support in the education-related literature for the need to establish clearer links between the local and the global in community environmental education programmes; the challenge was, as described by Sterling (1993: 80) how 'to be locally rooted with a planetary vision – community rather than insularity.'

But it is more than just about connecting, as Smith (1994: 16) quotes from the work of Geertz (1983) suggesting that local educators have to adopt the same mode of thinking, namely 'a continuous dialectical tacking between the most local of local detail and the most global of global structure in such a way as to bring them into simultaneous view.'

This linking of the local and global involves developing a broader understanding of environmental problems, which are often examined through a narrow scientific and technical perspective. A broader perspective requires a more holistic and integrated analysis of environmental problems that includes socioeconomic, political, cultural and historical contexts. Furthermore, there has been a trend in analysing environmental problems from the perspective of economic globalisation.

While this economic analysis is critical, it is equally important to establish links between the dynamic biophysical, social and political situations.

Progressive contextualisation as localisation therefore has a number of dimensions that are inter-related. In terms of the workshops the starting point was the local, that included the background and learning histories of the participants, the local environmental situation within a particular geographical space, and a more relational locality of shared characteristics across the participants or the space. However, it was critical to situate the local within the broader context, that is, the analysis of the environmental situation had to be informed by social, political, economic, cultural and historical contexts, as well as by establishing links between the local and the global situation.

Progressive Contextualisation as On-going

This practice of progressive contextualisation as localisation was primarily examined as a curriculum development process or what was earlier described as renewing RENEW. However, CEC-Phils experience of progressive contextualisation suggests this is not a one-way process. As shown in Figure 13.2 through the 'Contextualisation' and 'Transformation' arrows it was a reciprocal relationship between adapting educational practice to the local context, and the educational practice in turn contributing to transforming the local context. Furthermore, the on-going nature of this reciprocal process of progressive contextualisation, as represented by the middle spiral in Figure 13.2, resulted in an improvement of CEC-Phils education and organisational practice. The outermost spiral represents explicitly embedding progressive contextualisation within a research process. The resulting improvement of CEC's praxis is discussed below.

Three interdependent dimensions have been identified from CEC-Phils practice concerning the on-going and reciprocal nature of progressive contextualisation. Two dimensions involve outcomes of progressive contextualisation, namely; the on-going contextualisation that results in improved educational practice (not just the curriculum) and the resulting changed context. The third is a process dimension that has given added definition to the underlying action research approach integral to CEC's practice of progressive contextualisation.

The first outcome of progressive contextualisation highlights the need to constantly improve our own educational practice. This dimension relates to Paulo Freire's description that 'Education is thus constantly remade in the praxis. In order to be, it must become' (1993: 65). Freire established a critical connection between the on-going nature of the process and educational philosophy. He described that the 'banking method emphasises permanence and becomes reactionary,' on the other hand, 'a problem-posing education – which accepts neither a "well-behaved" present or a predetermined future – roots itself in the dynamic present and becomes revolutionary' (Freire 1993: 65).

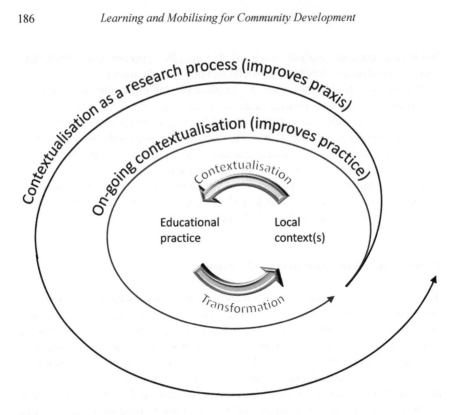

Figure 13.2   Progressive contextualisation as an on-going reciprocal process of transformation

The insight gained from the 'When do we start studying?' question posed by the sugar worker had very significant implications to our assumptions about effective teaching and learning approaches. While we still advocated for creative, participatory and experiential approaches to learning, we had to be more explicit about this approach at the start of the workshops. We did this by providing the participants with the opportunity to experience and reflect on their exposure to different ways of learning, and by introducing a participatory learning approach into the workshops.

The RENEW workshops were more interactive, which allowed us to use role play and simulations. For example, participants were assigned to role play different components of the environment to better illustrate the cyclical process of converting carbon dioxide to oxygen in photosynthesis, and oxygen to carbon dioxide in decomposition. The more technical CORETECH workshops would retain their interactive elements but with less fun activities and more hands-on learning. For example, a workshop on addressing the problem of golden apple snail infestation of rice fields, involved the farmers collecting snails at different stages in its life cycle to understand the impact of the government recommended pesticide on the snails and the health risks they posed on the farmers and their animals. In this particular instance, the pesticide killed the snails by dissolving their shells, which was also found to soften the hooves of animals and the toenails of the farmers.

Improvement was not limited to educational approaches but was also applied to the content of the RENEW workshops. The foundational concept of RENEW, the ecosystem concept, is explained as 'living and non-living elements of the environment that are interdependent on each other'. To facilitate the understanding of this concept, early RENEW workshops asked the participants to identify the different parts of their local environment through words, drawings, photos and so forth. This introductory activity allowed us to become more familiar with the components of the participants' local environment that could be used to illustrate the concepts of the workshop. After listing each of the components on a piece of paper, we asked the participants to classify the living and non-living things. In the past, this instruction had not posed any problem as the participants were generally able to distinguish parts of the environment that were living, like the plants, the animals, and the humans, and non-living parts, such as the air, the rocks and the water.

It was during a workshop conducted with indigenous groups from all over the Philippines that one participant asked, 'So what is non-living? Aren't all these components alive? The soil nurtures plants and the waters in the oceans provide us with fish. So what is non-living?' I paused. Thinking back to my own studies I realised that this particular knowledge had been gained from textbooks and that as an educator I had continued to pass on this knowledge to others. What the indigenous person had shared was his own knowledge and perspective about the environment he was familiar with. While the classification of living and non-living things is a foundational concept within science-orientated textbooks, it may not be fundamental to developing an understanding of the interconnections and interrelationships between the different parts of the environment.

My response to the participant was that while this classification is based on scientific thought, there are other ways of thinking about the environment, based on an understanding that all things are living and therefore need to be cared for. So instead of telling the indigenous person that he was wrong I introduced him to a knowledge system that provides information about how development project decisions are made and the effect they can have on the lives of individuals and communities, like his peoples.

Since that workshop, we no longer emphasise the concept of living and non-living things, rather we share this incident to help illustrate the different knowledge systems that exist. Learning about such knowledge systems helps us develop an appreciation of the different perspectives involved in environmental work.

This is a clear illustration of how educational practice (both in form and content) needs to be continuously re-created. Vargas (1997: 11) acknowledges both outcome dimensions by arguing that one of the challenges of popular education is ' .. more than just the revision of concepts [but] involves our capacity to adjust our practice to new contexts.'

The third dimension of the on-going nature of progressive contextualisation involves explicitly viewing this process as a research process, which results in the improvement of praxis (Figure 13.2). This is closely associated with the practice and principles of the reflective practitioner (Schön 1983), a particular stream within action research (Atweh, Kemmis and Weeks 1998).

Robottom and Hart (1993) describe a research situation very similar to the progressive contextualisation of CEC-Phils educational practice. 'There is a need, in participatory research in environmental education, for the methodology to be continually negotiated with participants as the substantive environmental and educational politics change and as joint understandings of the substantive issues and the relationships of the research to these issues become clearer' (Robottom and Hart 1993: 69).

This approach supports CEC-Phils initial experience of being mandated to develop baseline information on the state of the Philippines environment through a participatory grassroots research process. However, as discussed earlier, this approach proved difficult given the limited research capacities of the organisations that CEC-Phils worked with, and the lack of understanding and commitment to environmental work within the social movement for change. As such, an educational approach was adopted to equip the organisations and assist in developing their understanding of the environmental context of both organisations and communities they work with.

As illustrated in Table 13.1, the local environmental situation was one of the first modules within the RENEW workshops. Although this provided CEC-Phil with first-hand information from the participants it lacked a systematic approach to collating this information in order to develop a comprehensive picture of the Philippines environment. However, this local information did provide opportunities for on-going involvement of CEC-Phil with local organisations based on the environmental issues they were faced with. These opportunities were then harvested by the two other departments within CEC-Phils; the Research and the Networking Departments.

While there may have been a missed research opportunity due to the lack of systematic collection of stories shared during the RENEW workshops CEC-Phils had a strong culture of organisational reflection. In hindsight, these regular organisational processes facilitated not just the progressive contextualisation of our educational practice but also helped us to better appreciate and understand the on-going and reciprocal practice of progressive contextualisation.

Therefore, by identifying progressive contextualisation explicitly as a research process, informed by action research and the principles of reflective practice, it does not become merely a repetitive cyclical process of on-going and *ad hoc* adjustment. It helps to focus on progressive contextualisation as both an organisational and an educational process that develops a better understanding of the participants we work with, the contexts they live in and the appropriate actions to take within the broader framework of education leading to action and change. Making the action research dimension explicit also develops a better understanding of ourselves and our own educational practice.

Adapting and Transforming Context through Education

The EDSA People Power Revolution in 1986, as described in the Introduction of this book, provided the ground swell necessary to overthrow President Marcos. This event was the result of multiple contextual factors, complemented by many years of community-based organising, training and education, which are intimately interconnected in the Philippines. However, the overthrow of the Marcos regime did not result in the required systemic change of the socio-economic and political context.

This examination of CEC-Phils experience and practice of progressive contextualisation contributes to advancing the understanding and practice of education and training aimed at social change. Dynamic local and global contexts require that as community development workers and educators we are able to respond to transforming contexts. This chapter has identified the key factors that determine and shape this response. However, this chapter has also highlighted that as community development workers and educators, we cannot merely build the capacity of our communities to respond to these changes, in the name of community resilience. We need to work with our communities to develop their capacities to shape the factors that determine these changes. Therefore, the challenge to community-based educators and trainers is to continue to name the issues and identify the causes, as well as being able to build a curriculum that is responsive to the needs of the community. Furthermore, we cannot just solely design and deliver educational programmes that are responsive to context; the aim of our educational programmes is to contribute to challenging and transforming contexts.

To achieve these outcomes requires remaining open ourselves to being transformed through this educational process. This chapter has identified the reciprocal nature of progressive contextualisation, not just between the curriculum and the context, but in its capacity to transform how we and our organisations respond to and shape context.

The practice of progressive contextualisation was not a one-way process as I had originally anticipated, where the context shaped the education module. Guided by an action research approach, the process of curriculum development became an opportunity for CEC-Phil as an organisation to become both facilitator and an outcome of progressive contextualisation. We, the educators who were facilitating the process, were also outcomes of the process.

I did not realise how much meaning there was in my response to the sugarcane worker's question all those years ago when he asked, 'When do we start studying?'

'We have already started'.

References

Arquiza, Y. 1993. Green evolution: Nature groups fight over funds, principles. *Philippine Daily Inquirer*, 1 November, 6.

Atweh, B., Kemmis, S. and Weeks, P. 1998. *Action Research in Practice: Partnership for Social Justice in Education.* London: Routledge.

Coronel Ferrer, M. ed. 1997. *Civil Society Making Civil Society. Philippine Democracy Agenda: Volume 3.* Quezon City: Third World Studies Center: University of the Philippines.

Duhaylungsod, N. 1995. Preface in *Renewing RENEW: A Restoration Ecology Workshop Manual.* Quezon City: Center for Environmental Concerns-Philippines.

Duhaylungsod, N. 1998. A curricular development design for grassroots environmental education. *Watershed: Ideas on Environment and Society (Special Issue on Indigenous Knowledge Systems on Ecology Research),* 3(2), 9–14.

Freire, P. 1993. *Pedagogy of the Oppressed.* New York: Continuum.

Geertz, C. 1983. *Local Knowledge: Further Essays in Interpretive Anthropology.* New York: Basic Books.

Guevara, J.R. 1995. *Renewing RENEW: A Restoration Ecology Workshop Manual.* Quezon City: Center for Environmental Concerns-Philippines.

Guevara, J.R. 2002. *Popular Environmental Education: Progressive Contextualization of Local Practice in a Globalizing World.* Melbourne: Victoria University Unpublished PhD thesis.

Ife, J. 2002. *Community Development: Community-based Alternatives in an Age of Globalization.* New South Wales: Pearson Education.

Robottom, I. and Hart, P. 1993. *Research in Environmental Education: Engaging the Debate.* Geelong: Deakin-Griffith Environmental Education Project: Deakin University Press.

Schön, D.A. 1983. *The Reflective Practitioner: How Professionals Think in Action.* New York: Basic Books.

Smith, M. 1994. *Local Education: Community, Conversation, Praxis.* United Kingdom: Open University Press.

Sterling, S. 1993. A view from holistic ethics, in *Environmental Education: A Pathway to Sustainability,* edited by J. Fien. Geelong: Deakin University Press, 69–98.

Vargas, J.O. 1997. Rethinking popular education: An interim balance. *Adult Education and Development,* 48, 9–18.

Vayda, A. 1983. Progressive contextualization: Methods for research in human ecology. *Human Ecology,* 11(3), 265–81.

The World Bank. 1989. *Environment and Natural Resource Management Study, Volume 1.* Washington: The World Bank.

Chapter 14

The 'Craft' of Community-based Education and Training: The South African National Council of YMCAs and Youth Empowerment

Peter Westoby and Sipho Sokhela

Introduction

Young girls within South Africa are particularly vulnerable to teenage pregnancy and contracting HIV (Human Immunodeficiency Virus). For many initiatives aimed at changing this situation the key analysis is that young girls need information about reproductive health. The assumption is that information equals power – to have reproductive health information means to be empowered in negotiating sexuality. To a degree, this is true. However, this chapter describes and analyses an initiative that holds a deeper analysis: namely, that information alone does not equal power. Issues to do with HIV specifically and the girl-child's sexuality generally are embedded within relations of power that are about more than acquiring information.

At the heart of this chapter is a weaving of analysis around some of the challenges of initiating and maintaining a community-based education and training initiative that keeps issues of power central to its gaze and methods. It is posited that such a gaze requires an understanding of community-based training as craft. This community-based education and training initiative is a part of a peer education reproductive health programme in South Africa called the Better Life Options Program (BLP), run by the South African National Council of YMCAs (Young Men's Christian Associations). Furthermore, the chapter locates the work of community-based training within a broader framework of community development and social service delivery highlighting the different logics at work within each of them.

A Story of Community-based Training

Several years ago, one of the authors of this chapter was running a workshop for the BLP with the long-term, peer educators at a national conference in Cape

Town. The topic of that national conference was on boys' responsibilities within reproductive health issues.

During day one of the conference, several workshop activities focused on the key topic and by the end of the day all the peer educators appeared to have digested the 'content'. They could all verbally affirm with confidence that boys and young men should take more responsibility within sexual relationships around condom use and so forth. During the evening as the facilitator reflected on the day and planned the next he decided to try and 'test' the 'affirmations' and figured the best way would be to use a forum theatre technique (Boal 1979, Schutzman and Cohen-Cruz 1994: 2). He pulled aside a couple of the young people and quickly devised a script in which the two young people, now as actor and actress, would create a scene in which a young boy proceeded to seduce a young woman at home after a night out on the town. Within the acted scene the boy would offer the girl alcohol, which she accepted after a small amount of protest, and then they would fall into the flow of seduction, with her agreeing to have sex, and eventually, even agreeing to have sex without a condom, because firstly no one had a condom with them, and secondly, he insisted that he 'loved her'.

The next day the scene was acted in front of all the other peer educators with much laughter and delight. As per forum theatre methodology the facilitator then asked the two actors to restart the scene from the beginning and also invited spectators – more accurately named 'spect-actors' within forum theatre methodology (Schutzman and Cohen-Cruz 1994: 1) to call 'Stop!' at any time and come out and replace one of the actors. They could then continue to act out the scene as they saw fit and both 'spect-actors' would see if a different outcome could be achieved.

During the next twenty minutes or so, the scene was replayed about half a dozen times, usually still leading to the similar outcome of the young man sleeping with the young woman, although usually with a condom. However, what astounded the facilitator-trainer was that all replacements within the forum theatre process *replaced the girl*. In addition, this replaying usually attempted to negotiate a better outcome through modifying *her* behaviour (such as not accepting a drink in the first place), or being more assertive about her sexuality ('I will not sleep with you'), or being more resourceful ('I have a condom with me'). It should be said that with respect to the latter, usually having a condom with her was seen to be either 'sluttish' by the boy, turning him off from wanting sex with her (in the theatre scene that is), or irrelevant (that is, 'I do not use condoms').

After winding up the first stage of the forum theatre – six replacements of the girl – the trainer-facilitator referred back to the previous day's sessions about male responsibility within sexual relations and protection. Questions such as, 'What have you seen today?' and 'In what way does what you have seen relate to yesterday's workshop?' were asked. It was suggested that maybe the group should consider what relation those sessions might have to the forum-theatre experience. No one seemed to be able to 'connect the dots' and it was at this moment that the previous sense of being 'astounded' was reinforced with an intellectual curiosity about the now [failed] educational process initiated during day one.

The trainer-facilitator then asked the two initial actors to replay the scene and this time the trainer-facilitator himself called 'Stop!' and he *replaced the boy*. Moreover, this time the trainer-facilitator had a condom with him, and both actors agreed that if they were to have sex the male would want to use the condom. Again, spect-actors were asked, 'What do you see?'

The peer educators were now themselves astounded at both how 'easy' it was to change the outcome of the story (with both actors being happy and even being able to enjoy an alcoholic drink or two), and also at their own inability to have 'connected the dots' between the previous days' discussions about male responsibility and the actual attitudinal and behavioural change required. All that was needed was for someone to replace the male and take responsibility!

The trainer's educational curiosity remained. Reflecting on this 'ah-ha' moment in attempted transformational learning became a key motivator to consider the importance of firstly theatre, and other forms of embodied performative learning (Pettit 2010) within community-based training and secondly, the key role of the trainer as facilitator.

Clearly reflecting on this experience focuses on the failure of both orthodox educational practices, and even an embodied educational experience *as technique*. Neither the first days' learning nor the theatre experience would have led to transformational change within the context of gendered power relations, without the intervention of the facilitator. Recognition of this creates substantial challenges to thinking about initiating and maintaining community-based training processes that do keep power and transformation central to their gaze and analysis. However, before discussing this further we now step back to tell more about the story's context and programme.

The Context

The South African National Council of YMCAs is an indigenous membership-based youth organisation working throughout South Africa. It has approximately two thousand, five hundred members attached to both the National Council and 27 local 'branches' of YMCA located throughout the country. Since apartheid, the organisation like many within post-apartheid South Africa has been on an extraordinary journey of organisational transformation, reallocating resources and strategic priorities towards the historically disenfranchised black communities.

In 1994, one of the authors of this chapter was placed, through an Australian International Non-Government Organisation (INGO) called Australian Volunteers International, with the South African YMCA. The placement was with one of the YMCA's most progressive local branches on the South Coast of KwaZulu-Natal – managed and lead at that time by the other author of this chapter. The main focus of the local YMCA was a Supplementary Education Initiative (SEI) funded by AusAID through World Vision South Africa and World Vision Australia. This initiative was centred on providing a SEI educational *service* to young black South Africans at a period of incredible instability, with many black schools simply failing to function. The initiative also had an empowerment process, ensuring young people through locally formed committees, took control of the decision-making process of how the SEI projects would be developed, implemented and evaluated.

However, during the process of getting to know local young people through this service-delivery initiative a 'community analysis' (Westoby and Dowling 2009: 71ff) emerged. Both YMCA project staff and young people indicated that they felt something more substantial needed to be done about the growing teenage pregnancy rate and HIV/AIDS. In a sense a more *autonomous community development* process was emergent from the social service aspect of the project.

This was an historical period during which great stigma was associated with HIV, so most people would say that their friends were 'dying of TB' or some other associated illness. Participatory community-based research was initiated through the local YMCA youth networks in 1996 to find out about the knowledge, attitude and practices (KAP) of young people in relation to sexuality, protective behaviours, access to reproductive health services and so forth. This research provided a rationale to initiate some small educational initiatives within the structure of the SEI project that aimed to increase young people's knowledge of reproductive health.

Towards the end of 1996, several other INGOs had heard about the work of the YMCA on the South Coast of KwaZulu-Natal. One was a Washington, DC based organisation called the Centre for Development and Population Activities (CEDPA). A key reproductive health advocate, Seema Chauhan, visited the YMCAs and a process of partnership building was initiated with a view to 'scaling-up' some reproductive health interventions across the YMCA branches within South Africa, and eventually across the African Alliance Network of YMCAs.

The Community Education Initiative

Through listening to young people, bringing young people together and also working with the existing international experience of CEDPA generally, and Seema Chauhan particularly, the BLP was established within the South African YMCA. This programme targeted young girls as the key beneficiaries, and worked with young boys, parents, schools and other community leaders as key partners within the change process. The rationale for targeting the girl-child was their particular vulnerability when it came to firstly, [not] having information and knowledge about their sexuality and available services, and secondly, within the South African context it was incredibly difficult for young women to negotiate their sexuality within gendered relations of power and violence. That is, often boys, or worse still, groups of boys would not listen to a girl's assertion of 'No' in relation to her sexuality. Furthermore, our social analysis and research made it very clear that an underlying issue for many young women was economic, that is, their sexual selves were often the only bargaining power they had in negotiating many outcomes they wanted in relation to their life-goals.

At the heart of the BLP, and the key element relevant to the focus of this chapter, was the community-based peer education intervention that developed. Such peer education approaches are considered highly effective because peers have insider status and knowledge, and because the approach is participatory. Although there are many outstanding theoretical and practical issues in relation to understanding peer initiatives (Campbell and MacPhail 2002), peer education was in many ways the cornerstone of the BLP. This programme mobilised thousands of young people from late 1996 through to current times to educate their peers about their reproductive selves and reproductive rights. It also brought groups of young people together to tackle local issues of service provision; 'Where can I get condoms without everyone in the neighbourhood knowing?' or 'How can we band together to persuade the local police station to take rape seriously?'

The peer education intervention trained a pool of young girls as educators in reproductive health education issues and in facilitation skills, enabling them to then run small community-based training processes with other groups of young girls. The focus of these training processes was information as a mode of knowledge acquisition; skills development, such as assertiveness; and the development and implementation of local action plans around particular local concerns. The peer educators were provided with initial training, on-going supervision by a YMCA staff person, as well as regular extra training. Many of the peer educators also attended regular feedback workshops with YMCA staff and attended regional and national conferences, ensuring that they remained central to on-going design and redesign of training materials.

Locating the Community-based Education Work within a Broader Community Development and Service Delivery Framework

The threads of this story of work also helpfully illustrate how community-based education work can flow from, and sit within community development and social service delivery work. As community workers/writers we often find other practitioners wondering if they can sit one besides another. What we have learnt from this piece of work is that they can, as long as practitioners remain clear about which methodology is being used where, with clarity about the accompanying logics of each methodology. For example, within this work the SEI represents a *social service delivery* initiative, emergent from good consultation work with young people and communities, but ultimately developed out of a sense of national and donor priorities ('education for young people'). Initially the design of this project, by the YMCA, World Vision South Africa, World Vision Australia and AusAID had limited involvement of young people and communities within decision-making processes. The inclusion of youth committees as decision-making structures within the SEI was a change to the original design.

However, emergent from this social service delivery process was a *community development* process in which young people who, through the youth structures incorporated into the SEI, found their collective voice. As well as running the SEIs they identified their key priorities as dealing with teenage pregnancy and other reproductive health issues. They demanded changes to the SEI that initially incorporated reproductive health education workshops into the SEI curriculum. Furthermore, young people developed ideas and activities to address teenage pregnancy within their local communities – theatre at sports events, inclusion of information within community newspapers and so forth. As per orthodox community development work this initial work, thought about as just *activity*, soon required the formation of more carefully thought through *project* or community *programme* work, with the accompanying need for partnerships. At that stage, the YMCA who were driven less by staff-workers' agendas, and more by the young people's needs identification found that both CEDPA and the United Nations Population Fund (UNFPA), to be more than willing partners.

Despite this complex array of work, the key issue was that a social service oriented SEI project was now accompanied by a community development process *led by young people*, in partnership with YMCA workers and other organisational partners. Driven by young people, accompanied by such partners, a community-based education initiative was then developed in the form of a peer education strategy. The analysis emerging from the community development process was that a youth-led, peer education strategy, supported by community-based training of peer educators would be the most effective social change intervention in relation to reproductive health needs.

It is important to hold the three processes apart conceptually. These three processes include:

- the SEI *social service* programme – providing education services *for* young people
- the *youth-oriented community structure* (SEI committee) that could, through its new capacity develop young people's confidence, new skills, new relationships and networks, organisational partnerships, and initiate other community development initiatives as per emergent community analysis
- the BLP *community education* reproductive health initiative – working *with* young people, animated by young people through peer education.

The SEI continued for some five years and remained primarily a: (i) social service delivery intervention, albeit located effectively at community level. The SEI committee, while initially set up as a participatory structure for the SEI shifted towards holding a dual function. On one hand the committee continued to play the role of a *participatory* youth structure of the SEI, but on the other hand the committee now had changed into also being a: (ii) youth-oriented *community structure* in which young people could identify and initiate their own community-based initiatives. In this sense, it was the hub of youth-oriented community development processes that initiated new activities. Furthermore, one of the key community programmes emergent from this youth-oriented community structure was the: (iii) BLP with its focus on community education. Now we will refocus on the community education initiative itself.

Reflecting on the Story: Discussing Pedagogical and Programme Issues

Having described the context, the bare bones of the training intervention, and the conceptual understanding locating the intervention within a broader community development and social service framework we can return to the opening story and consider key pedagogical and programme issues. We have chosen to focus on how to maintain training around issues of power, not only information, and the 'trade-offs' in scaling-up community-based training work. Both areas are inter-twined.

Training around Issues of Power, not only Information

By situating the programme within an action learning framework we soon learnt, through reflecting on experiences such as the forum theatre described earlier, that community-based education focused on reproductive health/HIV *information* was not enough. In this case and context, information was not transformative. Young people acknowledged that they did not have enough correct information-knowledge about sexuality, their bodies, negotiating sex and so forth, yet it became quickly apparent that providing correct information-knowledge did not enable substantial change either. As mentioned above it became clear through on-going listening, feedback and learning from international good practice (Campbell and MacPhail 2002) that reproductive health issues are more related to issues of power – concerns of masculinity, gendered relations and economics rather than information.

Changes were made to the educational activities embedded within the peer education curricula ensuring that the programme was more focused on power issues – both analytically and in relation to skills learnt. For example, learning activities that helped young girls and young boys understand and deconstruct notions of sex and gender were incorporated. Discussions flowed from such activities enabling participants to understand what aspects of their lives were biologically determined and what were socially constructed. Particular exercises that enabled young people to draw and discuss what it is like to be a man or a woman in South Africa were elicited. For example, participants developed posters named 'Look like a man, act like a man' that depicted how young men's masculinities were culturally and socially constructed. Participants talked through how within popular constructions of femininity and masculinity conflict might be engaged-negotiated-resolved. Alternatives were then considered, particularly in relation to negotiating conflict around reproductive health that allowed people to practice their skills around conflict.

However, in acknowledging and understanding the importance of moving from information transmission focused on knowledge acquisition to transformational learning focused on issues of negotiating power, we also appreciate how easy it can be for practitioners and young peer education to revert to the former. Young people as peer educators, like many trainers, can resort, or more accurately reverse to the easy option of providing information. Despite all the modelling and mentoring around experientially and transformation-oriented facilitation the cultural and pedagogical pressure was towards reverting to education as information transfer.

This is hardly surprising when one considers the pedagogical emphasis of most marginalised educational contexts within South Africa. Young people, despite experiencing something 'dialogically different' within the YMCA training context, still also experience a predominant educational culture of what Paulo Freire (1970, 2006) called the 'banking model'. Daily many of the young people go to dysfunctional schools in which good practice is about teachers at least turning up for the day and delivering monological lessons. Thus transformational training goes very much 'against the grain'.

Coming to terms with this problem lead us to reflect on the challenges of facilitation for powerful transformation. Even if the issues discussed above can be dealt with, that is, reversing the cultural and pedagogical pressures towards information transmission, there is still the complex question of how to create and support facilitator training around complex issues such as power. What the introductory story illustrates is that moving from information-oriented to participatory and even embodied learning experiences does not guarantee transformative learning experiences, particularly if the goals are empowerment. Empowerment goals require facilitators who are equipped with both technique (including participatory or forum theatre techniques) and the ability to craft an 'ah-ha' moment. Such craft requires high-level consciousness, creativity, adaptability, discernment and insight.

The Trade-offs in Scaling-up such Community-based Training Processes

Such a conclusion leads to questions being asked about the quality of the work particularly in relation to trade-offs required by attempting to scale-up the work. For example, in scaling-up the work, to reach a much broader constituency of young people – given the scale of the challenge of HIV/AIDS and reproductive health rights – there is the need for, amongst others, *more*:

- professional staff to 'train' the young peer educators
- young people to be trained as peer educators
- involvement of local YMCA branches to manage the local initiatives
- co-ordination of the local initiatives, as per the nationally funded programme.

The emphasis on *more* signposts the issue of quantity. In this way scaling-up becomes a quantity issue that can at times conflict deeply with quality. There appear to be trade-offs required that at times are difficult to agree upon. Considering the introductory story and accompanying discussion above, an inherent tension exists between scaling-up the numbers of facilitators needed and ensuring all facilitators have understood the craft to work around issues of power and transformation.

Much can be learnt from Robert Chambers' reflections on similar challenges involving scaling-up participatory approaches to development. He argues that when thinking about scaling-up, 'Choices have to be made between working with initiatives and programmes which are small, slow and beautiful, and those which are big, fast and flawed' (Chambers 2005: 119). Chambers also argues that, 'Cases can be made for both. The best way forward may be slower than the speed demanded by sponsors [donors] but faster than the speed advocated by experienced field practitioners, with trade-offs between scale and speed, and quality' (2005: 119).

Certainly, tensions around such potential trade-offs were felt amongst practitioners within the YMCA BLP initiative. Whereas the initial small-scaled BLP initiative, developed within the SEI programme in KwaZulu-Natal, was made up of staff who had evolved with the programme learning skills and the craft on the job, the requirements of scaling-up necessitated finding staff through more orthodox ways of recruitment. Recruiting staff through advertising meant equipping them with (rather than evolving them through) transformational training craft, philosophy and techniques. What we learnt here was that it might be easy to equip people with the techniques, but not with the craft and philosophy of transformative training. This is because developing the craft and the philosophy is closely aligned with attitudes, consciousness and behaviours, and an overall commitment to empowerment. Staff training per se, finds it hard to 'develop' such a philosophy.

The trade-off is then between the qualities of trainers who can mobilise young people around an empowerment and transformational initiative versus the requirements of a quantity of trainers that can 'get the job done', meeting donor deadlines and outputs. Furthermore, the pressure of quantity leads to the development of a more manual-oriented training curricula, with heavily prescribed input/activities rather than menu-orientation where there is lots of flexibility within what facilitators chose to utilise. As core staff become less confident in the capacities of staff to train the young people *in situ* by drawing on a strong philosophy of empowerment, it then becomes easy to fall back on manuals – prescribing what should be done to peer educators to ensure they can deliver the group learning processes with other young people.

In some more serious ways, one of the key trade-offs seems to be the inherent challenge to peer education programmes. While the initial small-scale community-oriented peer programme was led by young people who had long affiliations' with the YMCA – their commitment to education was clear and credible – as the programme grew nationally young people became peer educators for more diverse reasons, of which some were not primarily about benefitting the key beneficiaries. Some young people became peer educators to gain skills for themselves, or access opportunities to travel to workshops in other parts of the country or region.

Having reflected on these experiences, and through the reading of literature around scaling-up, we propose that the key lessons learnt around scaling-up effective community-based training initiatives include:

- sticking to a flexible, trainer-friendly menu-oriented curricula rather than 'falling-back' upon a manual that prescribes what learning should take place
- scaling-up slowly, but persistently, driven not primarily by the agendas of donors, but by the agendas of demand from young people and communities (within the context of this story)
- the scaling-up process should be facilitated, not forced with the focus on trusting the local trainers and peer educators, rather than pre-determining targets that take precedence over process
- champions of change who have stuck with the community-based training work for some time and who with their historical memory ensure reflective capabilities and some level of continuity of learning
- drawing on Robert Chambers who advocates developing 'words and sayings' and 'stories' (2005: 149) to reflect the transformational heart of the work. For example, for many of the young girls participating in the programme the simple saying 'the gender agenda!' ensured they remained focused on what they had learnt about the social construction and deconstruction of relations between themselves and boys. Just as words and sayings used by facilitators such as 'hand over the pen' or 'hold your agenda lightly' remind trainers about process, the gender agenda constantly reminded people of key content issues relating to power and change
- to keep the community-based training programme 'on-track' requires the 'hosting' organisation to remain engaged in its own on-going transformational process ensuring there is a supportive action learning environment that fosters experimentation, risk-taking, honest reflection and change.

Conclusion

Initiating and sustaining community-based training initiatives that focus on power and individual and collective transformation-empowerment is incredibly difficult. At a micro-level, we have unpacked what could have easily ended as a failed training experience, despite our using strong participatory and embodied techniques. The conclusion reached is that the craft of facilitating transformational training is difficult to learn and not easily transmitted via most train-the-trainer programmes. The cultural and pedagogical pressure is towards informational transfer within initiatives such as the peer education Better Life Options Program. This pressure becomes even more pronounced when compounded by the need to achieve scale in order to inform large population groups about teenage pregnancy, HIV and reproductive health. Here, trade-offs between quantity and quality abound.

We propose that recognising the trade-offs, and therefore at times having to make tough pragmatic choices, needs to be accompanied by a deep commitment to ensuring facilitators of such community-based training are supported to learn the craft of transformative training. Philosophy and technique is not enough. It is the craft which is critical.

References

Boal, A. 1979. *Theatre of the Oppressed.* London: Pluto Press.

Campbell, C. and MacPhail, C. 2002. Peer education, gender and the development of critical consciousness: Participatory HIV prevention by South African youth. *Social Science and Medicine,* 55(2), 331–45.

Chambers, R. 2005. *Ideas for Development.* London: Earthscan.

Freire, P. 1970. *Pedagogy of the Oppressed.* New York: Continuum.

Freire, P. 2006. *Pedagogy of the Oppressed.* 30th Anniversary Edition. New York: Continuum.

Pettit, J. 2010. Multiple faces of power and learning. *IDS Bulletin, 41*(3), 25–35.

Schutzman, M. and Cohen-Cruz, J. eds 1994. *Playing Boal: Theatre, Therapy, Activism.* London: Routledge.

Westoby, P. and Dowling, G. 2009. *Dialogical Community Development: With Depth, Solidarity and Hospitality.* Brisbane: Tafina Press.

PART IV
Gathering the Wisdom from the Stories

Chapter 15

Conclusion: A Community-based Education and Training Framework

Lynda Shevellar and Peter Westoby

The stories within this book are stories about groups of people learning together and mobilising. As noted within the Introduction to this book, the collective of authors come from a diverse range of practice fields and disciplinary traditions – including community development, activism, feminism and conflict transformation. Their mobilising may be concerned with community building or it may be targeting direct action or resistance. The *content* of the learning is equally diverse: conflict resolution, environmental sustainability, and financial literacy, reproductive health, understanding social marginalisation, nonviolent action and so forth. What are common to all the stories are processes of community-based education and training – understood as social learning – that is integral to the group taking collective action, understood as mobilisation processes.

Within this conclusion, we want to pull some of the threads together and reflect on the processes of community-based education and training and collective social learning that lead to mobilisation. We have attempted to distil the diverse kinds of community-based education and training practices that have emerged from the stories; practices that are at times implicit and other times made explicit by the authors. In drawing upon the theory and stories that have been shared, our goal within this chapter is to construct a community-based education and training framework.

A framework is a conceptual structure that organises knowledge, philosophies, values and experience and names important dimensions of the work, so that practitioners can order their action. A framework assists community-based educators/trainers to organise their knowledge and experience of education and training, and furthermore to name important dimensions of their practice, enabling them to order the education and training practices. Our hunch from the beginning has been that by listening to and learning from the diverse stories we would be able to distil different education and training practices – and weave their common elements into a broader framework.

Our purpose in doing this is twofold. Firstly, it is to provide a framework for practitioners who might be working intuitively, or 'flying by the seat of their pants' so to speak. For such practitioners a framework might help them to be more disciplined or conscious in the work. Secondly, for practitioners who are already working with an education and training framework, we offer ours to initiate deeper reflection, and invite consideration of new practice wisdom.

A Note on the Method of Developing a Framework

As a process of developing this community-based education and training framework, we systematically followed the steps of building a framework as originally articulated by Kelly (Westoby and Ingamells 2011). The process required us to carefully read each of the stories of practice and distil key approaches. The many practices identified were thought of as data – and there was plenty of it with such a rich array of stories. Through discussion and reflection, our task was to then identify clusters of data that could be grouped into what is called a dimension. Our goal was to cluster the data into no more than seven dimensions, recognising that in practice trainers have to be able to remember the key dimensions, otherwise they do not help order and hold the work. Our next step was to consider how the dimensions related to each other – that is, to develop the structure of the framework. Our work of organising the data into dimensions and then shaping them is depicted in Figure 15.1.

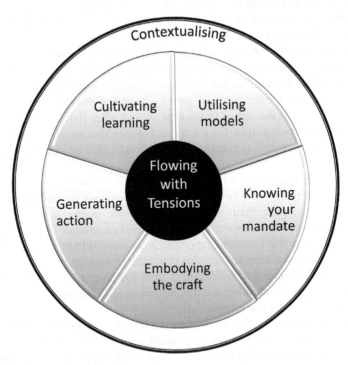

Figure 15.1　Dimensions of a community-based education and training framework

As can be seen, the structure of this framework is comprised of one central dimension: 'Flowing with tensions'; and one container dimension, that we name 'Contextualising'. There are then five additional dimensions that are to be held with equal weight and value. These include: utilising models, knowing your mandate, embodying the craft, generating action and cultivating learning. Finally, the steps of testing and critiquing the framework are the tasks for both authors and readers to do from here.

Each of the dimensions and the components of these, the sub-dimensions, are now discussed.

Dimension One: Flowing with Tensions

When considering the 12 stories of community-based education and training practice we were struck by the tensions embedded within the work. Examples of such tensions were between: facilitation and education; insider status and outsider status; information and empowerment; agenda driven training and participatory approaches; and action and learning. We felt that tension sat at the heart of every community-based education and training endeavour and was therefore the first dimension practitioners need to understand and work with.

In observing how people have handled tensions, we have been intrigued by how people work in ways that *hold* and *balance* tensions. These two verbs – hold and balance – are useful in that they help facilitators think about many of the paradoxes that are embedded in community-based education and training work, they also assist practitioners to not rush for resolution but to stay with the process. However, holding and balancing in our experience can also lead to people becoming stuck in paradox. Recognition of paradox is a rich moment in the learning process but it is not necessarily helpful in providing guidance within the action element of community-based education and training. Instead, we offer the idea of 'flowing with tensions' as a way of conceptualising the ability to move forward from a position of tension. It depicts the way in which educators/trainers have been able to engage with the identified tensions but have still been able to cultivate a movement – from paradox to clarity; from learning to action.

In this way, flowing with tensions has links to the work of psychologist Mihaly Csikszentmihalyi (1997), and his study of flow states. 'Flow' refers to a state of concentration or complete absorption. It is a state of being in which challenges are in balance with skills, and one becomes lost in an activity. Thus, the idea of flow contains a tension within itself: 'One has to be in control of the activity to experience it, yet one should not try to consciously control what one is doing' (Csikszentmihalyi 1999: 825). We see flowing with tensions as a similar absorption in activity, requiring not only skills and knowledge, but also an embodiment of the craft, discussed later in this conclusion. Flowing with tensions requires both mindfulness and surrender.

Finally, it is important to note that we have also chosen to locate this dimension at the centre of the framework because it relates to all of the other dimensions. As will be demonstrated below, there are many tensions embedded within knowing your mandate, utilising models, embodying the craft, generating action, cultivating learning and clarifying context and contextualisation. We hold flowing with tensions at the heart of our framework not only in acknowledgement of its pervasiveness within community-based learning, but also in recognition of its potential. This idea is perhaps best captured in the beautiful words of farmer, poet and academic, Wendell Berry, who says

> It may be that when we no longer know what to do we have come to our real work, and that when we no longer know which way to go we have begun our real journey. The mind that is not baffled is not employed. The impeded stream is the one that sings (Berry 1983: 97).

It is in flowing with tensions that our work 'sings'.

Dimension Two: Utilising Models

In reflecting on the different stories of practice, we were drawn to the clarity of models that were often being used. The second dimension of our framework therefore reminds educators/trainers to be conscious of the models available to guide their practice. Different models have different steps, as well as integrating elements of experience, new knowledge/theory, and application of knowledge in different ways. The key models we wish to summarise here in the conclusion are the experiential, elicitive, spiral, narrative and participatory learning and action models. This is not a definitive list of available models, but simply reflects those utilised most readily within this book. Although these can each be captured pictorially – as we have done below – we caution the over-reliance of such depictions. We are reminded of McTaggart's (1996) warning, that these representations are not a plea for slavish adherence to a procedure or recipe. Rather, such diagrams capture a series of commitments and principles, and depict the spirit as much as the method of engagement.

The Experiential Learning Model

This is shown in Figure 15.2, and is drawn from the work of David Kolb (1984). The experiential learning model involves (i) concrete experience followed by (ii) observation and reflection upon those experiences, followed by (iii) generalisations or the forming of abstract concepts based upon those reflections, and finally (iv) the application of those generalisations to new situations. The experiential learning cycle is discussed in the chapter by James Whelan et al, but is also implicit within many others. The training usually starts by drawing upon people's

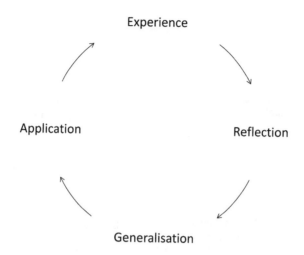

Figure 15.2   The experiential learning model

experience or by creating a new experience. The model is a spiral rather than a circle in that the four components of the action learning cycle keep repeating creating new and deeper experiences, reflections, generalisations and applications.

The Elicitive Model

This is shown most clearly in the chapters by Polly Walker and Howard Buckley, and begins with concrete experiences through a series of discovery-oriented activities (see Figure 15.3). Such activities are designed to act as catalysts for participants to *discover* what they do, and how they do it. Secondly, participants *name and categorise* the processes they use. Thirdly, participants engage in what Lederach (1995) refers to as 'contextualised *evaluation*'. In other words, once participants have a heightened awareness of what occurs in their situation they can examine it more objectively and consider the strengths and weaknesses of the approaches utilised. Fourthly, participants *re-create and adapt* their approaches, based on their evaluation. Finally, through either simulations or real-life experiences, participants try out their adapted models through *practical application*. One of the key differences between this and other models is that the elicitive model explicitly privileges culture (Lederach 1995). It is grounded in the view that culture and indigenous (or endogenous) knowledge is the 'seedbed' which gives rise to processes and models that better meet local needs.

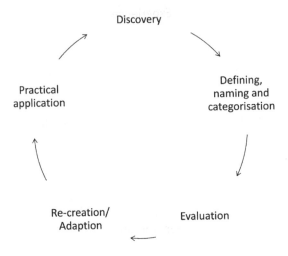

Figure 15.3   The elicitive model

The Spiral Model

This is shown in Figure 15.4, and is discussed most explicitly in the chapters by Alex Rayfield and Rennie Morello, and by Lynda Shevellar, Jane Sherwin and Gregory Mackay. The spiral model initially draws on the experiential learning cycle by inviting participants to reflect upon their experiences. Like the elicitive model, it seeks categorisations and pattern formation. However, the third step within the spiral model is what differentiates it, through the inclusion or insertion of new theory and information. The fourth step in the spiral model is to connect with the new knowledge, practice skills and to strategise and plan for action. Finally, the fifth step calls for applying strategies in action.

The Narrative Model

Figure 15.5, most obviously seen in the chapter by David Denborough, begins with individual experience through individual stories. It requires deep listening to enable the surfacing of common themes. Through these themes, individual accounts are woven together into a collective form. The reading and/or performing of the collective document then creates a new shared experience and builds a foundation for further learning and action.

The Participatory Learning and Action Model (PLA)

This is articulated clearly in Nicholas Haines's discussion about transformative learning in Cambodian farmer training. As Kumar observes (2002), while participatory processes are well known and employed regularly by facilitators,

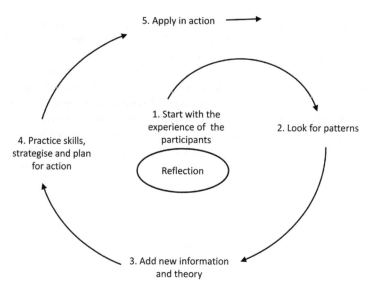

Source: Used with permission from Rick Arnold, Bev Burke, Carl James, D'Arcy Martin, and Barb Thomas. *Educating for a change*, Toronto: Between the Lines, 1991.

Figure 15.4   The spiral model

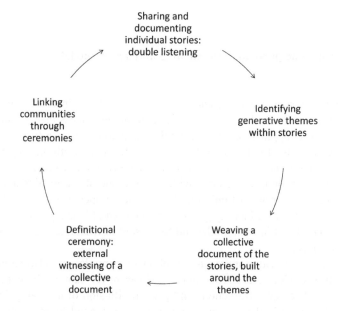

Figure 15.5   The narrative model

they tend to be relegated to a set of tools and techniques rather than understood in a broader framework for social action. For this reason, we choose to depart from the usual representations of PLA techniques and instead locate them within the broader spiral dynamic, as shown in Figure 15.6. We see participatory techniques (such as the use of community maps, charts, sociolines, photography, art, theatre and so forth) as a potent means of engaging with diversity, dynamics of power and creativity. In this way, they are tools upon which a powerful collective analysis can be built. As will be explored in dimension five, this analysis through reflection is not the endpoint, but the means by which action is designed, and agreement to act gained. Once action is taken, new opportunities for data collection emerge.

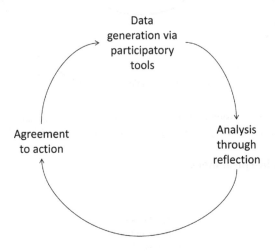

Figure 15.6   The participatory learning and action model

Each model presented here provides a systematic disciplined way of working with people's stories and experience, of integrating new ideas/theory and moving towards action or application. However, this dimension also needs to be understood within the previous discussion on flowing with tensions. Both our experience as educators/trainers and the stories of learning make clear that while it is very useful to enter an education/training space with a clear model it is critical to also be able to either let go of, or at least hold lightly, any model once it becomes a barrier to learning. Holding on and letting go captures the craft of being able to let go of the steps embedded within each model and be present to what might be happening in a learning space.

While we have written appreciatively about these models, we also acknowledge the limitations. Models are reductionist and can never capture the complexities of the work. They are abstractions and give the illusion of neutrality. However, as we will explore in the following dimensions, our mandate and context shape their application. Embedded in our discussion is an assumption about the capacity among facilitators for analysis, and among participants, a capacity for reflection. Yet recent work demonstrates that these are not simple skills, rather they are complex and difficult, requiring careful cultivation (Ryan 2011) and, as we will explore, to become embodied within our craft.

Dimension Three: Knowing your Mandate

Mandate is a reoccurring theme within the stories of practice, particularly when working within cross-cultural and post-colonial contexts. However, in our experience it is a key issue for all people entering a learning space. Briefly, knowing your mandate is a response to the perennial challenge of needing to know exactly *why* you are in a community setting conducting education and training, and/or needing to know what the 'content' area or objectives are within the learning process.

The question of why is ultimately a concern to do with legitimacy and authority: on whose authority is an educator/trainer resting when conducting an event? This can be a complex affair and often needs negotiating at multiple levels. For example, authority might be provided by an organisation seeking training, such as an INGO or government agency. But if the authority of that organisation is not accepted at a community level, then there will be little or no legitimacy of the training. In many ways, this negotiation of mandate requires the authority to be gained within a public space, whereas it might initially have been gained only in a private space. This kind of private negotiation occurs when an 'expert' asks a trainer to provide training to a group – possibly a private exchange between expert and trainer without involving the 'training beneficiaries'. To give the training real legitimacy there needs to be a process of gaining a public mandate, with the participants/potential beneficiaries, accepting that the process might lead to substantial change in relation to the training.

Furthermore, a mandate is needed to gain legitimacy in taking on particular education and training roles. For example, a facilitator may receive a mandate to 'provide' education or training in communication skills and may enter the space using an elicitive model. However, if over time, the facilitator recognises that provocation would help move the group forward, then a revised mandate would need to be sought to move into an emancipatory mode. This change in mandate can occur easily by asking a question such as, 'Do you give me permission to ask a hard question about how communication and power interact within your group?' Gaining that mandate makes it easier to enter the hard spaces that the group might not originally have expected to go.

Returning to the stories of this book, clearly gaining such a mandate becomes even more fraught when working cross-culturally. Polly Walker's story provides an honest and well-articulated account of this complexity – particularly in relation to issues such as gender. A group of male chiefs engaged in training might not provide initial legitimacy to a female trainer – the mandate to even conduct training therefore has not been negotiated. The chapter by Alex Rayfield and Rennie Morello raises questions about the mandate to train as outsiders and when not proficient in local people's language, therefore potentially reinforcing [neo] colonial relations.

Finally, mandate is critical in terms of the content of education and training. Who decides what should be included? Guides on participatory curriculum development (see Taylor 2003) provide useful practice wisdom about participants and key stakeholders designing the content areas they want to include within training. From our experience, this kind of participatory approach should be utilised within a dialogical ethos recognising that participants have a very good idea of their strengths and needs, but also recognising that educators/trainers have expertise that should be put on the table. As editors, we have particular memories where if a design process had been left completely to participants they would have crammed an enormous volume of material unrealistically into one workshop. In such a case, the trainers' expertise was essential in slowing down the content, creating time for reflection and linking to action. Community-based education and training while often participatory and emergent also needs to be content focused.

Dimension Four: Embodying the Craft

For our fourth dimension, we purposefully use the idea of craft as a way of capturing the technical elements of education and training alongside the imaginative and creative elements. An effective community-based practitioner needs to be both proficient in the techniques of education and training, as per any craftsperson, but also able to create a learning space using creativity and imagination. The idea of craft also alludes to being apprenticed, which is how many craftspeople learn their craft. In our experience effective trainers, good at their craft, have often been apprenticed to more experienced people – they learn alongside someone who gives them guidance and feedback.

The idea of embodying the craft alludes to educating and training with head, heart, hand, soul and body. All these elements of being human are needed within the learning space. The head brings analysis – of what to do, of what questions to ask. The heart brings a sense of care and discernment to the space – being able to know when it is time to push, let go and gentle people along. The hand brings a sense of practicality – getting on with writing or drawing on butchers paper or white boards. The soul brings depth and philosophy to the practice – being clear about goals, ideologies. And, the body brings senses into the space – unlocking learning as an embodied process that requires full engagement of the self, not just intellectual engagement. The chapter by Dave Andrews explicitly weaves together all of these elements. It shows intellectual rigour as the technical components of resourcing community work are considered, there is a deep emotional connection with people built on years of experience, there are spiritual and philosophical connections to the work guided by a sense of how we need to 'be' in the world, and there is ongoing action and a commitment to change. With this in mind, we now discuss several sub-dimensions of the crafting of the work, identified as key themes from the stories within this book.

The first is the art of questioning. Early in his career, Paulo Freire co-wrote a book with Antonio Faundez called *Learning to Question: A Pedagogy of Liberation* (1989). The title for us says it all – trainers need to learn to question. Effective community-based learning is often dependent on asking the right question at the right moment. Clearly each of the models discussed in dimension two lead to a different set of ordering of questions. Being clear about the question in the light of the model is critical. Often as facilitators, the key preparation required is taking the time to think about the questions that are going to be posed, with the hope that participants then ask their own questions. In creating a space of questioning, the quest for learning is animated.

The second sub-dimension of the craft is the centrality of stories and story-ing. Community-based education and training, as discussed in Chapter 1 of this book is about 'community' not as group-think, but as about a dialogue amongst individuals attempting to discern a common thread of analysis and agreement to act, and at the same time building a sense of themselves as a constituency. This dialogue is enabled through providing space for people to share or tell their personal stories related to the topic, issue or challenge at hand. The task of a community-based facilitator, again depending on the model of training, is to weave the individual stories together into, or discern with the participants what the public story is. The narrative training story, told by David Denborough, most clearly demonstrates this process through the creation of a collective public document, but many of the stories and models discussed in this book also require similar processes. Stories ground the training in people's real and identified concerns ensuring that the learning process and movement into action are public concerns of the group at hand.

Thirdly, we have identified embodied learning as a key sub-dimension of embodying the craft. By this, we refer to the several stories of practice that drew on forms of performance within the learning and action process. Kinds of performance discussed included song, participatory theatre and forum theatre. We, and our writing colleagues, are intrigued by the power of performance in enabling learning. Peter Westoby's and Sipho Sokhela's story of performance within reproductive health education within South Africa is particularly illustrative – not only of the power of performance, but again, and of significance to this discussion, the importance of the community-based educators/trainers craft in utilising such performance for emancipatory learning.

Fourthly, the name 'gentling' has been chosen to imagine the craft-work of pushing and pulling people within a training space (Westoby and Dowling 2009, Kelly forthcoming). There is acknowledgement that while an educator/trainer often invites people into a space of change – through learning and action – the invitation might also require what we think of as a gentle push or a pull. Freire and Horton talked about this as a 'delicate relationship' (Bell, Gaventa and Peters 1990). People's inertia of thought and body might create a sense of being stuck.

To push or pull people along is a process that requires discernment of where people are at and what they might be ready for. It requires moving people out of the comfort zone into the zone of discomfort (where real learning often takes place), without pushing them too far into a zone that lacks safety (where anxiety undermines any opportunity to learn) (King 2005). Gentling helps us imagine this process of pushing or pulling as something to be done with lightness and care. To push or pull comes with risk: people might respond positively and accompany the pushing or pulling, or they might resist. Imagining the craft of gentling ensures that the educator/trainer, as pusher or puller, moves with the response or reaction in a way that accompanies the people.

Fifthly, several of the stories within this book identify the importance of fun and humour within community-based education and training processes. Howard Buckley's reflection on Community Praxis Co-ops' experience of transformative leadership training is indicative of this importance. An educator/trainer needs to develop the craft of mixing the serious with the humorous, of discerning tension points that can be de-escalated through a joke, of deciding when to make light of heavy issues.

Sixthly, the craft of community-based education and training requires a capacity to hold or deal with conflict in ways that lead to generative rather than destructive outcomes for the group at hand. As should be clear to the reader by now, community-based education and training focuses on the collective process of learning *and* action and the collective emphasis requires strong skill-sets in holding and dealing with conflict. We use both words holding and dealing purposefully – the first as a way of identifying, sensing or 'singing up' conflicts that emerge within the group, and the second as a way of ensuring that they are not left to invisibly destroy a group process of learning and acting.

Finally, within this reflection on craft we have identified the sub-dimension of discernment. For us discernment feels like a kind of sixth sense that develops when involved in education and training over a long period of time. This sense is what enables an educator/trainer to recognise that something is not quite right – such as when Peter Westoby decided to use performance within the South African story. It could be thought of as a hunch, but develops through practice.

Dimension Five: Generating Action

Our fifth dimension, named as 'generating action' almost states the obvious. As we have already said, without action the learning experience may still be valuable and useful – but it is not community-based education and training. However, we have identified action as a dimension in acknowledgment that many people like to learn but do not want to act. It is more comfortable to remain in a learning space than to enter an active space. As educators and trainers, we often find we have to encourage and sometimes even push participants to act.

The generation of action is an essential element of all the stories in this book. Some action is easy to identify: such as the community projects and initiatives typically seen in community work. More radical work, such as that of Alex Rayfield and Rennie Morello and James Whelan et al, in direct action and civil resistance is the kind of action one might expect from community-based education and training. More subtly, for both David Denborough's healing work in Srebrenica and David Palmer's intergenerational work in the Kimberley, visits to place and story sharing were key components of the action. The work of Polly Walker, David Palmer and David Denborough all contained action as ceremonial elements that were in themselves both symbolic and transformative. In Kathy Landvogt's story of women and poverty in Melbourne, and in Peter Westoby and Sipho Sokhela's account of young people in South Africa, action took the form of community theatre, public performance and discussions, such as, 'What does it mean for us now moving from performance to the taking of responsibility around reproductive health?'

The distinction needs to be made between action and learning activities. Learning activities can be participatory, such as examining case studies, or participating in simulated events such as role play and skills rehearsal. However, by community action we mean that there is a direct movement from learning to action such that social change actually occurs. Consider Polly Walker's account of peace-building in Vanuatu, when she reflects: 'The previously aggrieved chiefs then said, 'It is finished; we are reconciled. Now we can begin the closing ceremony in peace. We can now say with truth that we are peacemakers.' The chiefs have not simply learnt processes for conflict resolution: they have experienced conflict resolution and through the learning processes they *have been reconciled*. Linking back to the first chapter of this book, and the distinction made between education and training, this helps explain why we argue that action is a key component of the training experience, and that the test of effective learning is action.

Dimension Six: Cultivating Learning

Dimension five critiqued the absence of learning without action. In this dimension, we caution against action without learning as unreflective action. At first, this dimension would seem self-explanatory. For this reason, we have named the dimension 'cultivating learning' because the *cultivation* of learning is the key. It is often the case that community organisers simply want an action to succeed, and this is encouraged by the age we are currently living in where time is equated with productivity and people are driven to fast decisions and instant gratification (see Agger 2004). On the other hand, as explored in the chapter by Lynda Shevellar, Jane Sherwin and Gregory Mackay mainstream educators tend to be more focused upon the learning as the outcome in itself. Community-based education and training seeks to fulfil both successful action and learning as necessary outcomes. This is what we mean by cultivation, and such cultivation is highly nuanced.

Cultivating learning requires us to resist the many myths surrounding education. The most damaging of myths is that of the individual learner: it is a Western image of the lone hero, making breakthroughs and jumps in wisdom in splendid isolation. Learning requires a multiplicity of experiences and knowledges and perspectives. Polly Walker's story of peace-building in Vanuatu speaks to the wisdom gained through co-learning. In her story, we see the delightful two-way movement of learning: co-learning occurs among participants, but it also occurs between facilitators and participants. Learning requires flowing through the tension of risk and safety. Such wisdom is apparent in the thinking of George Lakey who says 'to learn, people need to risk: to revise their conceptual framework, try a new skill, unlearn an old prejudice, admit there's something they don't know. To risk, people need safety. To be safe, they need a group and/or a teacher that supports them' (2010: 14).

George Lakey speaks of the role of the facilitator as being the creator of a 'container' for learning. And although ultimately people are responsible for their own learning, this does not mean the role of the facilitator is an easy one. The facilitator's role requires expertise in process, yet process that is open to change and movement. Facilitators may come with content knowledge, but need to exercise caution in the use of such expertise. They need to know where content knowledge sits in the learning process and how to hold back.

There is another dangerous myth – sadly spruiked too often to us in our academic roles – that those that cannot do: teach; and those that cannot teach: teach teachers! Our emphasis within this book on the cycles and spirals of learning are deliberate attempts to show that facilitating learning is complex, careful work. The chapter by Peter Westoby and Sipho Sokhela demonstrates how difficult this process can be. In their story of sex education with young people in South Africa, Peter and Sipho reflect on how people thought they had learnt, but the movement to discussions about action showed the gaps in their learning. If, as stated above, the test of effective learning is action, we can now add to this that the test of good action is its emergence from learning.

Dimension Seven: Contextualising

We have named the seventh dimension 'contextualising' to reflect the wisdom embraced by many of the stories within this book. These stories demonstrate that understanding, engaging and transforming context is critical for fruitful community-based education and training efforts. We have purposefully named it as a verb – contextualis*ing* – in an attempt to focus on the dynamic, on-going and adaptive element of the dimension. Contextualising does *not* signpost a process of conducting some pre-research to gain understanding of a context within which a community practitioner will be operating. Instead it signposts the need to cultivate an attitude of shifting education and training practices in the light of constantly trying to understand complex shifting contexts, AND holding onto the notion that community-based education and training, as a process of learning and action, can contribute to the shifting or transformation of context.

Context was often brought to the fore at some point within the chapters. Practitioners clearly had developed a much-nuanced understanding of historical, cultural, political and social contexts, whether they were in South Africa, Vanuatu, West Papua, the Philippines or Brisbane. However, what was striking for us as editors/authors was the dynamic and engaged nature of that understanding. Polly Walker's story of the work in Vanuatu is foremost in identifying the cultural dimension of such contextualising, acknowledging and arguing for a deep understanding of how worldviews are shaping peoples understanding of their context, thereby acknowledging that education and training practices need to be relevant to such worldviews, but also recognising that the processes could shift worldviews. Jose Robbie Guevara's reflections on his work within the Philippines are most clear about identifying contextualisation as a central element to any community-based education or training efforts. For him it is an on-going cyclical process requiring educational and training practices to be constantly contextualised to the local situation, thereby ensuring that the relevant educational and training practices can be truly transformational. To not contextualise is to ensure that the practices remain surface oriented, not rooted deeply within the local and therefore unable to transform the context. This is the essence of it – contextualising ensures that community-based educators and trainers not only adapt their practices to context, but also ensure their practices lead to actions that transform context.

Conclusion

The framework and the associated dimensions discussed above could be construed as the outcome of an action research cycle of the book's editors attempting to make sense of 12 stories of community-based education and training practice. Each story was filled with wisdom. We have attempted to distil some of that wisdom and weave it together into a framework that can now be utilised by many practitioners. As such, it is a framework that we think and hope is rooted in real-world community practice, one not divorced from the complexities of such settings. As such, it is a theory-building exercise, thinking of theory as a lens of sense-making. The framework as a theory of practice assists the community development practitioner to think about conducting education and training. The next step is theory-testing, inviting practitioners to use the framework and then reflect on its [in]adequacies, its strengths and limitations. We invite practitioners to do that and to continue the dialogue with us.

References

Agger, B. 2004. *Speeding Up Fast Capitalism: Cultures, Jobs, Families, Schools, Bodies.* Colarado: Paradigm Publishers.

Bell, B. Gaventa, J. and Peters, J. eds 1990. *We Make the Road by Walking: Conversations on Education and Social Change: Myles Horton and Paulo Freire.* Philadelphia: Temple University Press.

Berry, W. 1983. Poetry and marriage, in *Standing by Words: Essays.* California: Counterpoint Press, 92–105.

Csikszentmihalyi, M. 1997. *Finding Flow: The Psychology of Engagement with Everyday Life.* New York: Basic Books.

Csikszentmihalyi, M. 1999. If we are so rich, why aren't we happy? *American Psychologist,* 54(10), 821–7.

Freire, P. and Faundez, A. 1989. *Learning to Question: A Pedagogy of Liberation.* Geneva: WCC Publications.

Kelly, A., forthcoming. *With Love and a Sense of Necessity.*

King, K. 2005. *Bringing Transformative Learning to Life.* Florida: Kreiger Publishing Company.

Kolb, D.A. 1984. *Experiential Learning: Experience as the Source of Learning and Development.* Englewood Cliffs: Prentice Hall.

Kumar, S. 2002. *Methods for Community Participation: A Complete Guide for Practitioners.* London: ITDG Publishing.

Lakey, G. 2010. *Facilitating Group Learning: Strategies for Success with Diverse Adult Learners.* San Francisco: Jossey Bass.

Lederach, J.P. 1995. *Preparing For Peace: Conflict Transformation Across Cultures.* New York: Syracuse University Press.

McTaggart, R. 1996. Issues for participatory action researchers, in *New Directions in Action Research,* edited by O. Zuber-Skerritt. London: The Falmer Press, 243–55.

Ryan, M. 2011. Improving reflective writing in higher education: A social semiotic perspective. *Teaching in Higher Education,* 16(1), 99–111.

Taylor, P. 2003. *How to Design a Training Course: A Guide to Participatory Curriculum Development.* New York: Continuum.

Westoby, P. and Dowling, G. 2009. *Dialogical Community Development: With Depth Solidarity and Hospitality.* Brisbane: Tafina Press.

Westoby, P. and Ingamells, A. 2011. Teaching community development personal practice frameworks. *Social Work Education*[Online: 23 February]. Available at: (iFirst), 1–14. doi: 10.1080/02615479.2010.550913 [accessed: 22 March 2011].

Index

For Product Safety Concerns and Information please contact our
EU representative GPSR@taylorandfrancis.com Taylor & Francis
Verlag GmbH, Kaufingerstraße 24, 80331 München, Germany